101

HEART

HEALTHY

Lifestyles

Simple ways, based on scientific evidence, to prevent, delay the onset of, slow the progression of, or even reverse

heart disease

First Edition

Disclaimer

This book summarizes information on the role of lifestyles in health and illness. Readers should be aware that knowledge of medicine is constantly evolving. This book is not intended as a substitute for the medical advice of your physicians or other trained health care professional.

Do not disregard professional medical advice or delay seeking it because of something you have read in this book. Do not embark on any lifestyle change without seeking your health care provider's advice. It is a clinicians' responsibility, relying on their experience and knowledge of their patients, to determine the best plan of care, including lifestyle change advice.

Reviewing or following information contained in this book, does not constitute a physician-patient relationship. The authors and publisher accept no liability for any injury arising out of the use of material contained herein, and make no warranty, express or implied, with respect to the contents of this publication.

To you, the reader.

Wishing you a healthier, happier, and longer life.

CONTENTS

PREFACE

Cardiovascular disease is the number one killer worldwide. The data shows that globally (in 2013), 31 percent of all deaths were a result of cardiovascular diseases, with 80 percent of these deaths occurring in low- and middle-income countries. Stroke accounted for 11.8 percent of these deaths. Cardiovascular disease is also a major killer in the United States of America. According to the latest statistics released by the American Heart Association (in 2013) cardiovascular diseases claimed 801,000 lives. Of these, heart disease killed more than 370,000 people and strokes killed nearly 129,000 people. Cardiovascular diseases are even more dangerous in the African-American population - 48 percent of women and 46 percent of men have some form of cardiovascular disease. According to the American Heart Association, about 2,200 Americans die of cardiovascular disease each day - an average of 1 death every 40 seconds. It is estimated that you have one in three chances of dying from cardiovascular disease.

Arterial atherosclerosis is the major underlying pathology behind heart attacks and strokes – the most common of all cardiovascular diseases. Low grade vascular inflammation appears to be the initiating factor - leading to the development of atherosclerosis. A recent study, called CANTOS, appears to confirm that reducing inflammation is associated with a reduction in atherosclerosis and major cardiovascular events.[1] Inflammation causes endothelial (the inner lining of blood vessels) dysfunction, allowing low-density lipoprotein cholesterol in your blood to infiltrate this lining, where they get oxidized. The immune system sends over macrophages, which swallow these oxidized low-density cholesterol particles. The macrophages get loaded with fat – and become 'foam cells'. These fat laden cells continue to accumulate inside the arterial wall – this is atherosclerosis. Because of this continuing infilteration, the arterial walls become thick and less elastic. As the foam cells grow in volume, the collection ultimately encroaches the inner lumen of the artery, forming a plaque. The covering wall of the plaque may rupture and open a wound inside the artery. This wound sets into motion a cascade of events – platelets and clotting proteins rush to this area to heal the wound by forming a blood clot. This unfortunately cuts off the blood supply further down – resulting in a heart attack (damaged or dead heart muscle) or stroke (damaged or dead brain tissue). These events often occur suddenly and may be fatal. Throughout this book you will read words such as anti-inflammation, lipid lowering, anti-oxidant, anti-vasospasm, anti-platelet, anti-aggregation and mention of blood clotting proteins such as reduction in fibrinogen. These actions are beneficial and help prevent or reduce the atherosclerotic process and the resultant major events such as heart attacks or strokes. A large amount of scientific data has clearly identified major life factors that increase inflammation and raise the risk of getting cardiovascular diseases. Many of these factors are based on our lifestyles and are fortunately modifiable.

The recommendations are not based on our opinion alone. Everything suggested in this book has been proven by large, well structured, scientific studies, done at major centers all over the world, under the supervision of well renowned medical scientists. These studies have been replicated repeatedly and the benefits of these interventions verified objectively. We have selected only a few studies in each chapter, to impress upon you the cardiovascular benefit stemming from incorporating that particular lifestyle.

We have also included some data on some medications, supplements and diseases that deleteriously affect the heart. Although not strictly lifestyle changes, the information provided will help you be aware of the cardiovascular dangers associated with these. This way you may be able to make better lifestyle choices. We have aslo included a chapter on height – a short height increases your risk of coronary heart disease when compared to taller people and is a non-modifiable factor. However, our reason for including it in this book is to advise you that if you are relatively short, you should be even more diligent in making healthy lifestyle changes. Further, all the information in this book is evidence based, and there are many difficult medical terms. We have therefore attached a glossary towards the end. Finally, new studies with new data are always coming in. The advise we give today may be stale tomorrow or even proven to be wrong. For example, a recent report from a study called PURE, is suggesting that eating saturated fat in moderation may be actually good for you.[2] So please keep your knowledge updated.

This book presents you with recommendations for healthy life-style interventions, based on scientific evidence. Incorporating lifestyle changes gradually, you may not only live a healthier and better life, but increase your disability free life span by several years. This extra life could be as high as 12 years in women and 11 years in men.[3] And it will not only cost you less for staying healthy, but like the old cliché says, 'health is wealth', potentially extend your earning years. Imagine the love and happiness that you and your loved ones will experience with you growing old gracefully and in good health.

Please heed our advice, but make sure your health provider is aware of any changes you make in your lifestyles and is in agreement with your decision. Incorporate these simple life-style interventions gradually. But start immediately. We only wish you to have a happy and healthy long life – a life not marred by the worry of cardiovascular disease. Wish you all the best in this healthy adventure.

Neil K. Agarwal, MD

Internal Medicine

Shashi K. Agarwal, MD

Cardiovascular Diseases

References

1. Canakinumab Anti-inflammatory Thrombosis Outcomes Study (CANTOS): https://www.escardio.org/The-ESC/Press-Office/Press-releases/drug-cuts-cardiovascular-disease-and-lung-cancer-risk-by-reducing-inflammation-cantos. Accessed September, 13 2017.
2. Prospective Urban Rural Epidemiology (PURE) Study: https://www.escardio.org/The-ESC/Press-Office/Press-releases/revisiting-dietary-fat-guidelines-pure. Accessed September, 13, 2017.
3. Neil Mehta, Mikko Myrskyl&#2013265924;. The Population Health Benefits Of A Healthy Lifestyle: Life Expectancy Increased And Onset Of Disability Delayed. Health Affairs, 2017; 10.1377/hlthaff.2016.1569 DOI: 10.1377/hlthaff.2016.1569. Accessed September 13, 2017.

1. ALCOHOL

Introduction

Drinking an alcoholic beverage is a common social practice in many parts of the world. The active ingredient is ethanol. Imbibed in small to moderate doses, it reduces anxiety and increases the ease of socialization. In small to moderate doses there is an associated euphoria, while at higher doses it causes intoxication, and may result in unconsciousness and even death. Drinking alcohol is not new – fermented drinks were consumed as early as the Neolithic period.[1] Common fermented alcoholic drinks are beer, wine, cider and mead, while common distilled drinks are whiskey, vodka and brandy. Gin is a purified spirit. In general, the alcohol by volume is 5% in beers, 13.5% in wines, 30%-40% in spirits and 4% -8% in cider. The amount of alcohol in a standard drink in the United States, is 0.6 oz. (18 ml). A standard drink may be considered approximately a 12 oz. (350 ml) glass of beer, 8-9 oz. of malt liquor, a 5 oz. (150 ml) glass of wine, 3-4 oz. of fortified wine, 2-3 oz. of a cordial, a 1.5 oz. (44 ml) glass of a 80 US proof spirit or a 1 oz. of 100-proof spirits. Drinking mild to moderate amounts of alcohol have been found to be heart protective.

Scientific Evidence

- Several epidemiologic and clinical studies have demonstrated the protective effects of moderate alcohol intake on the heart.[2-5]
- Researchers from the University of Calgary, University of Texas Health Science Center, and Harvard Medical School identified 4,235 studies dealing with the effects of alcohol on the cardiovascular system. These studies included more than two million men and women who were followed for an average of 11 years. They concluded that when compared with no alcohol use, moderate alcohol use reduced the risk of a new diagnosis of coronary artery disease by 29%; reduced the risk of dying from any cardiovascular disease by 25%; reduced the risk of dying from a heart attack or coronary artery disease by 25%; reduced the risk of dying from any cause by 13% and reduced the risk of having an ischemic (clot-caused) stroke by 8%. There was however an increase in the risk of having a hemorrhagic (bleeding) stroke by 14%.[6]

- Alcohol protects the cardiovascular system in many ways. These include raising the protective high-density lipoprotein cholesterol (the 'good cholesterol') and decreasing the harmful oxidation of the low-density lipoprotein cholesterol (the 'bad' cholesterol). It also decreases the levels of fibrinogen, thereby protecting against blood clots. There is decreased tendency for platelets to aggregate and there is an increased blood flow to the heart.[7,8]

Conclusion

Mild to moderate alcohol drinking is cardioprotective. Most major health societies recommend that if you drink, do so in moderation. This means an average of one to two drinks per day for men and one drink per day for women. (A drink is one 12 oz. beer, 4 oz. of wine, 1.5 oz. of 80-proof spirits, or 1 oz. of 100-proof spirits.) Drinking in moderation will provide you with many other health benefits, including a decreased risk of developing diabetes mellitus.[9] Exceeding the recommended limits may cause serious health problems, including elevated blood triglycerides, high blood pressure, obesity, and heart failure. Binge drinking can also lead to a stroke. Other serious cardiovascular conditions that excessive alcohol can cause include cardiomyopathy, cardiac arrhythmia and sudden cardiac death.[10]

Lifestyle Implications

Drinking one to two alcoholic drinks per day for men and one alcoholic drink per day for women, is cardioprotective. Do not drink alcohol if pregnant.

References

1. https://en.wikipedia.org/wiki/Alcoholic_drink
2. Colditz GA, Branch LG, Lipnick RJ, Willett WC, Rosner B, Posner B, et al. Moderate alcohol and decreased cardiovascular mortality in an elderly cohort. Am Heart J 1985;109:886-9.
3. Camargo CA, Hennekens CH, Gaziano JM, Glynn RJ, Manson JE, Stampfer MJ. Prospective study of moderate alcohol consumption and mortality in US male physicians. Arch Intern Med 1997;157:79-85.
4. Berger K, Ajani UA, Kase CS, Gaziano JM, Buring JE, Glynn RJ, et al. Light-to-moderate alcohol consumption and risk of stroke among US male physicians. N Engl J Med 1999;341:1557-64.

5. Djousse L, Lee IM, Buring JE, Gaziano JM. Alcohol consumption and risk of cardiovascular disease and death in women: potential mediating mechanisms. Circulation 2009;120:237-44.

6. Ronksley Paul E, Brien Susan E, Turner Barbara J, Mukamal Kenneth J, Ghali William A. Association of alcohol consumption with selected cardiovascular disease outcomes: a systematic review and meta-analysis BMJ 2011; 342: d671.

7. Ginter E, Simko V. Ethanol and cardiovascular diseases: epidemiological, biochemical and clinical aspects. Bratisl Lek Listy. 2008;109:590–594.

8. Collins MA, Neafsey EJ, Mukamal KJ, Gray MO, Parks DA, Das DK, Korthuis RJ. Alcohol in moderation, cardioprotection, and neuroprotection: epidemiological considerations and mechanistic studies. Alcohol Clin Exp Res. 2009;33:206–219.

9. Lando L.J. Koppes, Jacqueline M. Dekker, Henk F.J. Hendriks, Lex M. Bouter, Robert J. Heine. Moderate Alcohol Consumption Lowers the Risk of Type 2 Diabetes. Diabetes Care Mar 2005, 28 (3) 719-725.

10. http://www.heart.org/HEARTORG/HealthyLiving/HealthyEating/Nutrition/Alcohol-and-Heart-Health_UCM_305173_Article.jsp#.WYEzSYjys1I

2. ANGER

Introduction

The emotion of anger has been studied by scholars over several centuries. Galen and Seneca regarded anger as a kind of madness. Over the centuries several experts have voiced their opinions regarding anger. Several religions also view anger as a negative trait (Judaism), a deadly sin (Christianity) instigated by the devil (Islam) or a result of ignorance. (Hinduism). Anger, an intense emotional reaction, can be both constructive (problem solving) and destructive (self-justification and assigning blame elsewhere; holding grudges and intensifying long term animosity). Anger, especially the destructive kind, stimulates the hypothalamic–pituitary–adrenal axis and precipitates increased levels of adrenaline and noradrenaline – resulting in physical responses such as an increased heart rate and elevated blood pressure, which are detrimental to the cardiovascular system. Several recent studies have reported data confirming the scientific co-relation between anger and coronary artery disease and elevated cardiovascular morbidity and mortality. The catecholamines released by anger also lead to narrowing of the coronary arteries in diseased areas and a reduction in the amount of blood pumped by the heart.[1]

Scientific Evidence

- The Framingham Heart Study in 1980 reported that suppressed anger independently predicted the 8-year incidence of coronary heart disease among both men and women.[2]
- In a 3-year follow-up study of 3750 Finnish men aged 40 to 59, high ratings of hostility in men with preexisting heart disease were associated with an increased coronary heart disease mortality.[3]
- Men with a high potential for hostility, studied in the Multiple Risk Factor Intervention Trial, had a 50% higher risk of coronary heart disease.[4]
- Episodes of anger were 2.3 times more likely to trigger a heart attack in the Determinants of Myocardial Infarction Onset Study.[5]
- The Normative Aging Study examined whether problems controlling one's anger would predict coronary heart disease events among men. These prospective data, based on a study of a total of

1305 men, suggest that anger is associated with a twofold to threefold increase in the risk of total coronary heart disease and angina pectoris.[6]

- Anger induces a multitude of neurological and vascular changes, resulting in the discharge of circulating catecholamines, increased myocardial oxygen demand, and increased platelet aggregability.[7]
- Several recent publications have re-confirmed the negative association between anger and coronary heart disease.[8]

Conclusion

Anger is a common emotion, but a low threshold for anger, excessive anger or suppressed and retained anger induces neuro-vascular changes in the human body resulting in increased narrowing of the coronary arteries, especially if already diseased, and an increased propensity for blood clot formation, which may result in a complete blockage of the blood flow in these vessels – causing a heart attack. The result is an increased coronary heart disease morbidity and mortality. Proactively raising the threshold for proneness to and decreasing the intensity of the eruption of anger emotions may be achieved by psychological self-training or external help. This may help your cardiovascular system last longer.

Lifestyle Implications

Excessive or suppressed anger is a dangerous emotion for your heart.

References

1. Boltwood MD, Taylor CB, Boutte Burke M, Grogin H, Giacomini J. Anger report predicts coronary artery vasomotor response to mental stress in atherosclerotic segments. Am J Cardiol. 1993;72:1361-1365.
2. Haynes SG, Feinleib M, Kannel WB. The relationship of psychosocial factors to coronary heart disease in the Framingham study, III: Eight-year incidence of coronary heart disease. Am J Epidemiol. 1980 Jan;111(1):37-58.
3. Koskenvuo M, Kaprio J, Rose RJ, Kesaniemi A, Sarna S, Heikkila K, Langinvainio H. Hostility as a risk factor for mortality and ischemic heart disease in men. Psychosom Med. 1988;50:153-164.
4. Dembroski TM, MacDougall JM, Costa PT Jr, Grandits GA. Components of hostility as predictors of sudden death and myocardial infarction in the Multiple Risk Factor Intervention Trial. Psychosom Med. 1989;51:514-522.

5.   Dembroski TM, MacDougall JM, Costa PT Jr, Grandits GA. Components of Mittleman MA, Maclure M, Sherwood JB, et al. Triggering of acute myocardial infarction onset by episodes of anger. Circulation. 1995;92:1720-1725.

6.   Kawachi I, Sparrow D, Spiro A III, Vokonas P, Weiss ST. A prospective study of anger and coronary heart disease: the Normative Aging Study. Circulation. 1996;94:2090–2095

7.   Verrier RL, Hagestad EL, Lown B. Delayed myocardial ischemia induced by anger. Circulation. 1987;75:249-254.

8.   Thomas Buckley, Soon Y Soo Hoo, Judith Fethney et al. Triggering of acute coronary occlusion by episodes of anger. European Heart Journal: Acute Cardiovascular Care. Vol 4, Issue 6, 2015, page(s): 493-498

3. ANTIOXIDANTS

Introduction

Antioxidants are found in many foods, especially fruits and vegetables. They include beta-carotene, lutein, lycopene, selenium and vitamins A, C and E. Antioxidants counteract oxidative stress. Reduced endogenous anti-oxidants or an excessive pro-oxidant production, as seen in diabetes, hyperlipidemia, hypertension, and obesity leads to increased atherosclerosis and coronary heart disease.[1] Oxidative stress may also be increased by several environmental factors such as smoking, second hand tobacco smoke,[2] and pollution.[3] Oxidative stress results in endothelial dysfunction. It also activates inflammation, immune responses, and thrombus formation. It oxidizes lipids - these events lead to the development of atherosclerosis — the main pathology behind coronary heart disease.[4] Fruits and vegetables are high in anti-oxidants and their increased consumption decreases cardiovascular disease. However, oral anti-oxidant supplementation does not provide the same benefit.

Scientific Evidence

- A Cochrane review (Cochrane Reviews are internationally recognized as the highest standard in evidence-based health care.) of the impact of antioxidant supplements on healthy individuals (26 trials), or in people with one or more of a range of diseases (52 trials), including cardiovascular disease (10 trials), found no overall reduction in all-cause mortality, irrespective of the combination of antioxidants used.[5]
- In a review of 68 randomized trials with 232 606 participants, it was found that some antioxidants (β-carotene, vitamin A, and vitamin E) have the potential to increase mortality, either singly or when combined with other antioxidant supplements. Vitamin A increased mortality by 16%, beta carotene increased mortality by 5%, and vitamin E increased mortality by 4%.[6]

Conclusion

Antioxidants are extremely helpful in protecting against oxidative stress, which leads to oxidation of the 'bad' low density lipoprotein cholesterol, a major event leading to the development of atherosclerosis. However, only natural foods rich in anti-oxidants appear to confer this benefit. Most clinical studies have not replicated the benefits using anti-oxidant supplements. As a matter of fact, some antioxidants (β-carotene, vitamin A, and vitamin E) taken as supplements appear to increase mortality.

Lifestyle Implications

The cardiovascular benefits of antioxidant supplementation have yet to be proven. The best antioxidants for cardiovascular protection are obtained via an increased intake of fruits and vegetables.

References

1. West IC. Radicals and oxidative stress in diabetes. Diabet Med (2000) 17(3):171–80.
2. Bernhard D, Wang XL. Smoking, oxidative stress and cardiovascular diseases – do anti-oxidative therapies fail? Curr Med Chem (2007) 14(16):1703–12.10.2174/092986707781058959.
3. Newby DE, Mannucci PM, Tell GS, Baccarelli AA, Brook RD, Donaldson K, et al. Expert position paper on air pollution and cardiovascular disease. Eur Heart J (2015) 36(2):83–93.10.1093/eurheartj/ehu458.
4. Le Brocq M, Leslie SJ, Milliken P, Megson IL. Endothelial dysfunction: from molecular mechanisms to measurement, clinical implications, and therapeutic opportunities. Antioxid Redox Signal (2008) 10(9):1631–74.10.1089/ars.2007.2013.
5. Bjelakovic G, Nikolova D, Gluud LL, Simonetti RG, Gluud C. Antioxidant supplements for prevention of mortality in healthy participants and patients with various diseases. Cochrane Database Syst Rev (2012) 3:CD007176.10.1002/14651858.CD007470.pub2.
6. Bjelakovic G, Nikolova D, Gluud L, et al. Mortality in randomized trials of antioxidant supplements for primary and secondary prevention. Systematic review and meta-analysis. Journal of the American Medical Association. 2007;297:842-857.

4. ANXIETY

Introduction

Anxiety, usually in response to stressful situations, is occasionally experienced by most human beings. This form of anxiety is just one color in our emotional rainbow. However, protracted, severe or worsening anxiety can cause both emotional and physical harm. Persistent anxiety is a pathological psychiatric diagnosis – generalized anxiety disorder. Anxiety often accompanies depression and is also an important component of panic attacks and obsessive-compulsive disorder. Fear of social situations is often due to a social anxiety disorder. Anxiety may also play a major role in post-traumatic stress disorder. Anxiety initiates cardiovascular responses such as a rapid heart rate, increased blood pressure and decreased heart rate variability. These are all conducive to development or aggravation of cardiovascular diseases, especially coronary heart disease.[1] Several recent articles have reviewed the negative association between anxiety and cardiovascular disease.[2] In a recent report by Berge and associates, the risk for ischemic heart disease in persons with high levels of anxiety is increased by about 70%.[3]

Scientific Evidence

- Psychological factors such as anxiety and depression negatively impact cardiovascular diseases.[4,5]
- A meta-analysis of twenty studies involving 249,846 persons with a mean follow-up period of 11.2 years for incident coronary heart disease was done. Researchers found that anxiety was an independent risk factor for incident coronary heart disease and cardiac mortality. The risk of coronary heart disease and cardiac death was increased by 26% and 48% respectively in anxious people.[6]
- In a survey of 49,321 young Swedish men, 18 to 20 years of age, who were medically examined for military service in 1969 and 1970, the diagnosis of anxiety independently predicted subsequent coronary heart disease events.[7]
- Preexisting depression and anxiety also predict future hospitalizations in patients with established cardiovascular disease.[8]

- Post-traumatic stress disorder is a high anxiety disorder due to exposure to traumatic events. In this meta-analysis, researchers found that post-traumatic stress disorder appears to impart a twofold risk of recurrent acute coronary syndrome.[9]
- In another meta-analysis, generalized anxiety disorder was associated with a 21 % increase in the risk of sustaining a major adverse cardiac event.[10]
- Recent studies have confirmed repeatedly the deleterious effects of anxiety on ischemic heart disease. The risk for ischemic heart disease in persons with high levels of anxiety is increased by about 70%.[3]

Conclusion

Anxiety comes in several forms in daily life. However, beware of high levels of anxiety as it will damage your cardiovascular system. There are several treatment regimens for controlling excessive anxiety and include anxiety management through relaxation exercises, sensory focusing, and yoga exercises. Cognitive restructuring to prevent catastrophizing and gradual and repeated exposure to the fearsome environment to ease the anxiety, is also beneficial.

Lifestyle Implications

Relax. Your heart will thank you.

References

1. http://www.hopkinsmedicine.org/heart_vascular_institute/clinical_servic es/centers_excellence/womens_cardiovascular_health_center/patient_inf ormation/health_topics/anxiety_heart_disease.html
2. Cohen BE, Edmondson D, Kronish IM. State of the Art Review: Depression, Stress, Anxiety, and Cardiovascular Disease. American Journal of Hypertension. 2015;28(11):1295-1302.
3. Berge LI, Skogen JC, Sulo G, et al. Health anxiety and risk of ischaemic heart disease: a prospective cohort study linking the Hordaland Health Study (HUSK) with the Cardiovascular Diseases in Norway (CVDNOR) project. BMJ Open. 2016;6(11): e012914.
4. Rozanski A, Blumenthal JA, Kaplan J. Impact of psychological factors on the pathogenesis of cardiovascular disease and implications for therapy. Circulation. 1999;99(16):2192-2217
5. Everson-Rose SA, Lewis TT. Psychosocial factors and cardiovascular diseases. Annu Rev Public Health. 2005;26:469-500.

6. Roest AM, Martens EJ, de Jonge P, Denollet J. Anxiety and risk of incident coronary heart disease: a meta-analysis. J Am Coll Cardiol. 2010;56(1): 38-46.

7. Janszky I, Ahnve S, Lundberg I, Hemmingsson T. Early-onset depression, anxiety, and risk of subsequent coronary heart disease: 37-year follow-up of 49,321 young Swedish men. J Am Coll Cardiol. 2010;56(1):31-37.

8. Chamberlain AM, Vickers KS, Colligan RC, et al. Associations of Preexisting Depression and Anxiety with Hospitalization in Patients with Cardiovascular Disease. Mayo Clinic Proceedings. 2011;86(11):1056-1062.

9. Edmondson D, Richardson S, Falzon L, et al. Posttraumatic stress disorder prevalence and risk of recurrence in acute coronary syndrome patients: a meta-analytic review. PLoS ONE. 2012;7:e38915.

10. Tully PJ, Cosh SM, Baumeister H. The anxious heart in whose mind? A systematic review and meta-regression of factors associated with anxiety disorder diagnosis, treatment and morbidity risk in coronary heart disease. J Psychosom Res. 2014;77:439–48.

5. AROMATHERAPY

Introduction

Essential oils are obtained by steam distillation of aromatic plants. Controlled use of these essential oils is aromatherapy ("aroma" meaning a pleasant scent and "therapy" meaning healing). These fragrant essential oils are absorbed into the human body through airway or the skin.[1] It is estimated that approximately 4.5% of American adults use some form of complementary medicine to help them sleep, and this includes aromatherapy.[2] Neroli oil and Lavender oil are commonly used in controlling insomnia. Aromatherapy is also used for borderline hypertension. Common essential oils used in the treatment of high blood pressure include lavender (*Lavandula officinalis*), marjoram (*Origanum majorana*), ylang-ylang (*Cananga odorata*), and Neroli (*Citrus aurantium*). Lemon (*Citrus limon*), Clary sage (*Salvia sclarea*) and Rose (*Rosa damascene, Rosa centifolia*). Essential oils appear to modulate the autonomic nervous system by reducing the sympathetic activity and increasing the parasympathetic activity and thereby reducing blood pressure. Aromatherapy with Lavender, Roman chamomile (*Chamaemelum nobile*) and Rose also helps induce relaxation, which reduces fear and anxiety associated with a myocardial infarction or cardiovascular surgery.

Scientific Evidence

- A study investigating the effects of aroma massage (using a blend of lavender, ylang-ylang, marjoram, and Neroli) showed an approximate reduction of 15 mmHg for home systolic blood pressure, while the placebo group showed an approximate reduction of only 6 mmHg.[3]
- In another study, reductions in blood pressure (average 4.70/1.21 mm Hg after inhalation) were associated with a decrease in the salivary cortisol levels in 83 prehypertensive and hypertensive subjects.[4] Inhalation of essential oil appears to be more effective in reducing the stress hormone cortisol.[5]
- Aromatherapy with essential oils blended with lavender, roman chamomile, and neroli in a ratio of 6 : 2 : 0.5 helped reduce the

anxiety levels and increased the sleep quality of percutaneous coronary intervention patients admitted to the intensive care unit.[6]

- The result of another study showed that inhaling pure lavender extract for 20-30 minutes is effective in reducing anxiety and blood pressure on heart attack patients hospitalized in the coronary care unit.[7]
- Inadequate or improper sleep is also a risk factor for cardiovascular disease. This has been well documented in nursing shift workers. Aromatherapy has been found in several studies to improve sleep quality in people.[8-10]

Conclusion

The data on aromatherapy and protection against cardiovascular diseases is soft. However, the relaxing effects of aromatherapy should provide a 'feel good' atmosphere and calm the sympathetic nervous system. Essential oils are easily available, cheap and easy to apply. Relaxation therapy using essential oils in the form of inhalation from a necklace may be worth trying, especially if you have prehypertension or borderline hypertension. Essential oil can also be massaged or placed as drops on the pillow before going to sleep.

Lifestyle Implications

A good relaxing sleep with aromatherapy can be good for your blood pressure.

References

1. Su C. Y. Aromatherapy and health care. Science Development. 2012;469:26–31.
2. NCCAM Health Information. Aromatherapy. 2010.
3. Ju M-S, Lee S, Bae I, Hur M-H, Seong K, Lee MS. Effects of Aroma Massage on Home Blood Pressure, Ambulatory Blood Pressure, and Sleep Quality in Middle-Aged Women with Hypertension. Evidence-based Complementary and Alternative Medicine: eCAM. 2013;2013:403251.
4. Kim I-H, Kim C, Seong K, Hur M-H, Lim HM, Lee MS. Essential Oil Inhalation on Blood Pressure and Salivary Cortisol Levels in Prehypertensive and Hypertensive Subjects. Evidence-based Complementary and Alternative Medicine : eCAM. 2012;2012:984203.
5. Kim JS. Effects of the aromatherapy on stress related hormone. Department of Nursing, Keimyung University, Daegu, Korea, 2007.

6. Mi-Yeon Cho, Eun Sil Min, Myung-Haeng Hur, and Myeong Soo Lee. Effects of Aromatherapy on the Anxiety, Vital Signs, and Sleep Quality of Percutaneous Coronary Intervention Patients in Intensive Care Units. Evidence-Based Complementary and Alternative Medicine, Volume 2013, Article ID 381381, 6 pages.

7. Mirbastegan Na, Ganjloo Jb, Bakhshandeh Bavarsad Mc, Rakhshani MHd Effects of Aromatherapy on Anxiety and Vital Signs ofMyocardial Infarction Patients in Intensive Care Units. IMJM Volume 15 Number 2, Dec 2016.

8. Shimada K., Fukuda S., Maeda K., et al. Aromatherapy alleviates endothelial dysfunction of medical staff after night-shift work: preliminary observations. Hypertension Research. 2011;34(2):264–267.

9. Yazdi Z., Sadeghniiat-Haghighi K., Javadi A. R. H. S., Rikhtegar G. Sleep quality and insomnia in nurses with different circadian chronotypes: morningness and eveningness orientation. Work. 2014;47(4):561–567.

10. Chang Y-Y, Lin C-L, Chang L-Y. The Effects of Aromatherapy Massage on Sleep Quality of Nurses on Monthly Rotating Night Shifts. Evidence-based Complementary and Alternative Medicine : eCAM. 2017;2017:3861273.

6. ASPIRIN

Introduction

Hippocrates recognized the pain and fever relieving properties of the willow leaves around 460 to 377 B.C. However, the benefit of willow bark extract in reducing fever, pain and inflammation was only formally investigated in the mid-eighteenth century. Salicylic acid, the active compound of willow extract, led to the formulation of a stable form of acetylsalicylic acid - the modern-day aspirin. Dr. Felix Hoffmann achieved this feat at the Bayer laboratories in Leverkusen on 10 August, 1897. The name was derived from "a" for acetyl, "spir" from Spiraea, and "in" as a common ending for a drug. Aspirin was marketed in 1899 by Bayer. Today, aspirin is a widely used medication all over the world. It is estimated that 40,000 tons (50 to 120 billion pills) are consumed each year worldwide. Dosage may vary from 75 mg to 500 mg, with many strengths in between. The standard low dose aspirin contains 81 mg and regular aspirin contains 325 mg. Prophylactic aspirin is beneficial in reducing the risks of heart disease and colorectal cancer, in some groups of people.

Scientific Evidence

- Baigent and associates performed a meta-analysis of serious vascular events and major bleeds in six primary prevention trials (95,000 individuals at low-average risk, 660,000 person-years, 3,554 serious vascular events) and 16 secondary prevention trials (17,000 individuals at high-average risk, 43,000 person-years, 3,306 serious vascular events) that compared long-term low dose aspirin versus control.[1] They found that aspirin reduced the incidence of cardiovascular events by 12%, both in the general population and in high-risk groups.

- Several meta-analyses indicate that in individuals at low risk for cardiovascular disease, aspirin reduces the risk of myocardial infarction, but there is an increase in major bleeding.[2] The European Society of Cardiology recommends that low-dose aspirin for primary cardiovascular prevention be used in patients at high cardiovascular risk, defined as ≥ 2 major cardiovascular events (death, myocardial infarction, or stroke) projected per 100 person-years, who are not at increased risk of bleeding.[3]

- In 2016, the US Preventive Services Task Force recommended initiating low dose aspirin for the primary prevention of both cardiovascular disease and colorectal cancer among adults ages 50 to 59 who are at increased risk for cardiovascular disease. Adults 60 to 69 who are at increased cardiovascular disease risk may also benefit. They also cautioned that harms may exceed benefits for persons starting aspirin in their 70s.[4]

- In several cardiovascular disease primary prevention studies, there was a 58% increased risk of major gastrointestinal bleeding and a 27% increased risk of hemorrhagic stroke in patients taking very-low-dose aspirin ($\leq$100 mg daily or every other day) Aspirin, even in low doses, is not benign and should be used only according to the recommendations.[5]

- For secondary prevention in patients with established coronary artery disease, low dose aspirin should be taken for 1-year post-acute coronary syndrome, with prior revascularization, coronary stenosis > 50% by coronary angiogram, and/or evidence for cardiac ischemia on diagnostic testing. In the first-year post-acute coronary syndrome, low dose aspirin is usually combined with other anti-platelet agents.[6]

Conclusion

Aspirin is available over the counter and taking aspirin for pain, fever or inflammation is almost a normal lifestyle phenomenon. It is therefore included as a lifestyle choice. Low dose aspirin may help in both primary and secondary prevention of ischemic heart disease. However, it increases the risk of gastrointestinal and intracranial bleeding. Therefore, we recommend you follow advice from your healthcare provider.

Lifestyle Implications

A baby aspirin a day may be cardiovascular protective but take it only after clearance from your health care provider.

References

1. Baigent C, Blackwell L, Collins R, et al. Aspirin in the primary and secondary prevention of vascular disease: collaborative meta-analysis of individual participant data from randomised trials. Lancet. 2009;373:1849–1860.

2.   Raju NC, Eikelboom JW. The aspirin controversy in primary prevention. Curr Opin Cardiol. 2012 Sep;27(5):499-507

3.   Halvorsen S, Andreotti F, ten Berg JM, et al. Aspirin therapy in primary cardiovascular disease prevention: a position paper of the European Society of Cardiology working group on thrombosis. J Am Coll Cardiol. 2014 Jul 22;64(3):319-27

4.   Dehmer SP, Maciosek MV, Flottemesch TJ, et al. Aspirin for the Primary Prevention of Cardiovascular Disease and Colorectal Cancer: A Decision Analysis for the U.S. Preventive Services Task Force. Ann Intern Med. 2016 Jun 21;164(12):777-86.

5.   Whitlock EP, Burda BU, Williams SB, et al. Bleeding Risks with Aspirin Use for Primary Prevention in Adults: A Systematic Review for the U.S. Preventive Services Task Force. Ann Intern Med. 2016 Jun 21;164(12):826-35.

6.   Vandvik PO, Lincoff AM, Gore JM, et al. Primary and Secondary Prevention of Cardiovascular Disease: Antithrombotic Therapy and Prevention of Thrombosis, 9th ed: American College of Chest Physicians Evidence-Based Clinical Practice Guidelines. Chest. 2012;141(2 Suppl): e637S-e668S.

7. BERRIES

Introduction

Fruits and vegetables are universally accepted as being cardiovascular healthy.[1] Berries are fruits with strong bioactive compounds and are often referred to as super foods or functional foods. The commonly consumed berries in the United States include blackberry, raspberry, blueberry, cranberry, and strawberries. Less commonly consumed berries include acai, black currant, chokeberry, and mulberries. Berries are low in calories and are high in moisture and fiber.[2] They are high in phytochemicals, especially anthocyanins. They also have strong anti-oxidant properties. Besides the anthocyanins, berries are also rich in many other beneficial chemicals. These phytochemicals include flavonols, tannins, and phenolic acids. Berries are healthy for the cardiovascular system.[3]

Scientific Evidence

- **Blackberry** *(Rubus fruticosus):* A 100 gm serving of blackberries contains 43 calories and 25% of the daily value of fiber and vitamin C and 19% daily value of vitamin K. Blackberry seeds contain oils rich in omega-3 and omga-6 fats and contain numerous cardiovascular protective phytochemicals and fiber.[4] Blackberries possess diverse pharmacological activities, including antioxidant properties, which make them cardioprotective.[5]
- **Blueberry** *(Vaccinium corymbosum)*: Blueberries are a good source of fiber, vitamin C, and are rich in anthocyanidin antioxidants.[6] They exhibit bioactive activities that include antioxidant, anti-inflammation, and anti-angiogenesis effects. Blueberries help prevent several age-related chronic diseases affecting the cardiovascular system such as diabetes, hyperlipidemia, obesity and atherosclerosis.[7]
- **Cranberry** *(Vaccinium macrocarpon)*: Cranberries are rich in Vitamin C and several phenolic compounds. Cranberry juice has been extensively studied for therapeutic benefits in several diseases including diabetes, metabolic syndrome, obesity, and cardiovascular disease.[8]
- **Red raspberry** *(Rubus idaeus)*: Red raspberries are rich in vitamin C, fiber, manganese and antioxidant phytochemicals, especially

anthocyanins and ellagitannins. Studies indicate significant
antioxidant activity. They also demonstrate antidiabetic and
antihypertensive effects.[9]

- **Strawberry** *(Fragaria x ananassa):* Strawberries are a rich source of
  sugars, vitamins (ascorbic acid and folate), and minerals, as well as
  bioactive compounds such as flavonoids, anthocyanins and
  phenolic acids. Strawberries attenuate oxidative stress and
  inflammation, hyperglycemia and hyperlipidemia and metabolic
  syndrome.[10] Strawberries are heart healthy.

Other berries, although less commonly consumed, also have several
cardioprotective effects.

Conclusion

Berries derive their rich dark colors from anti-oxidant anthocyanin
pigments. They also exert many other beneficial effects that positively
impact the cardiovascular system. The most commonly consumed berries
have significant cardiovascular protective effects.

Lifestyle Implications

*Eat richly colored berries regularly. They can be eaten raw or mixed in salads or added to
fruit juice.*

References

1. Joanne L. Slavin, and Beate Lloyd. Health Benefits of Fruits and
   Vegetables. Adv Nutr July 2012 Adv Nutr vol. 3: 506-516.
2. Basu A, Rhone M, Lyons TJ. Berries: emerging impact on cardiovascular
   health. *Nutrition reviews.* 2010;68(3):168-177.
3. Rissanen TH, Voutilainen S, Virtanen JK, et al. Low intake of fruits,
   berries and vegetables is associated with excess mortality in men: the
   Kuopio Ischaemic Heart Disease Risk Factor (KIHD) Study. J
   Nutr. 2003;133:199–204.
4. Sellappan, S.; Akoh, C. C.; Krewer, G. "Phenolic compounds and
   antioxidant capacity of Georgia-grown blueberries and blackberries".
   Journal of Agricultural and Food Chemistry. 2002, 50 (8): 2432–2438.
5. Dai J, Patel JD, Mumper RJ. Characterization of blackberry extract and its
   antiproliferative and anti-inflammatory properties. J Med Food. 2007 Jun;
   10(2):258-65.
6. de Souza VR, Pereira PA, da Silva TL, de Oliveira Lima LC, Pio R,
   Queiroz F. Determination of the bioactive compounds, antioxidant
   activity and chemical composition of Brazilian blackberry, red raspberry,

strawberry, blueberry and sweet cherry fruits. Food Chem. 2014 Aug 1;
156:362-8.

7. Wu X, Kang J, Xie C, Burris R, Ferguson ME, Badger TM, Nagarajan S.
Dietary blueberries attenuate atherosclerosis in apolipoprotein E-deficient
mice by upregulating antioxidant enzyme expression. J Nutr. 2010 Sep;
140(9):1628-32.

8. Shidfar F, Heydari, Hajimiresmaiel SJ, Hosseini S, Shidfar S, Amiri F. The
effects of cranberry juice on serum glucose, apoB, apoA-I, Lp(a), and
Paraoxonase-1 activity in type 2 diabetic male patients. J Res Med Sci.
2012 Apr;17(4):355-60.

9. Cheplick S., Kwon Y., Bhowmik P., Shetty K. Clonal variation in
raspberry fruit phenolics and relevance for diabetes and hypertension
management. J. Food Biochem. 2007;31: 656–679.

10. Basu A, Fu DX, Wilkinson M, Simmons B, Wu M, Betts NM, Du M,
Lyons TJ. Strawberries decrease atherosclerotic markers in subjects with
metabolic syndrome. Nutr Res. 2010 Jul;30(7):462-9.

8. BINGE DRINKING

Introduction

Drinking alcohol is a common social pastime in the United States. Drinking in moderation has cardiovascular protective effects - an average of one to two drinks per day for men and one drink per day for non-pregnant women. The amount of alcohol in a standard drink in the United States, is 0.6 US fluid ounces (18 ml). A standard drink may be considered approximately a 12 oz. (350 ml) glass of beer, 8-9 oz. of malt liquor, a 5 oz. (150 ml) glass of wine, 3-4 oz. of fortified wine, 2-3 oz. of a cordial, a 1.5 oz. (44 ml) glass of a 40% ABV (80 US proof) spirit or a 1 oz. of 100-proof spirits. However, excessive drinking (for men, 15 or more drinks per week and for women, 8 or more drinks per week) has significant harmful effects including accidental injuries, violence, risky sexual behaviors, high blood pressure, stroke, several cancers, liver and digestive diseases and mental health problems. Binge drinking, the most common form of excessive drinking, is defined as consuming 5 or more drinks for men and 4 or more drinks for women, during a single occasion.[1] Binge drinking is associated with a higher cardiovascular risk.

Scientific Evidence

- In a study of 3,869 participants from the Determinants of Myocardial Infarction Onset Study, the incidence rate of acute myocardial infarction onset was elevated 1.72-fold within 1 hour after alcohol consumption.[2] In this study, gin, vodka and whiskey drinkers were at the greatest risk and those who drank beer and wine were at a lesser risk.
- In a review of 14 studies containing 4,718 ischemic heart disease events (morbidity and mortality), researchers found that the pooled relative risk of a major cardiovascular event. in irregular heavy drinking compared with regular moderate drinking was 1.45 (45% higher in the former). This indicates that when light to moderate drinking is mixed with occasional heavy drinking, the cardioprotective effect of moderate alcohol consumption disappears.[3]
- A prospective cohort study done over a period of ten years involving 15,965 Finnish men and women aged 25 to 64 years,

found that binge drinkers had almost double the risk for ischemic stroke when compared to non-binge drinkers.[4]

- Alcohol also may induce cardiac arrhythmias. At the 2015 Munich Octoberfest, 3,028 voluntary participants were monitored for breath alcohol concentration and cardiac arrhythmias. Cardiac arrhythmias occurred in 30.5% (sinus tachycardia 25.9%; other arrhythmia subtypes 5.4%) and correlated with the breath alcohol concentration. Autonomic imbalance is probably behind this phenomenon.[5]

- In the 1999-2002 National Health and Nutrition Examination Survey of current drinkers aged 20-84 year without cardiovascular disease, binge drinking once per week or more, increased the risk of developing metabolic syndrome by 51%.[6] Metabolic syndrome is a significant risk factor for cardiovascular diseases.

Conclusion

Alcohol is a double-edged sword. Drinking in moderation provides significant cardiovascular protection while drinking in excess is associated with a litany of dangerous cardiac problems. Binge drinking, consuming 5 or more drinks for men and 4 or more drinks for women, during a single occasion is also dangerous, especially in the short term. The dangers appear more in non-regular drinkers. So, follow the recommendations and stay away from excessive drinking – it is safer for the cardiovascular system.

Lifestyle Implications

Drink alcohol in moderation (one to two alcoholic drinks per day for men and one alcoholic drink per day for women). Binge drinking is dangerous and can kill you.

References

1. https://www.cdc.gov/alcohol/fact-sheets/alcohol-use.htm
2. Mostofsky, Elizabetha, van der Bom, et al. Risk of Myocardial Infarction Immediately After Alcohol Consumption. Epidemiology: March 2015 - Volume 26 - Issue 2 - p 143–150.
3. Roerecke M, Rehm J (2010) Irregular heavy drinking occasions and risk of ischemic heart disease: a systematic review and meta-analysis. Am J Epidemiol 171: 633–644.
4. Sundell L, Salomaa V, Vartiainen E, Poikolainen K, Laatikainen T (2008) Increased stroke risk is related to a binge-drinking habit. Stroke 39: 3179–3184.

5.   Brunner S, Herbel R, Drobesch C, Peters A, Massberg S, Kääb S, Sinner MF. Alcohol consumption, sinus tachycardia, and cardiac arrhythmias at the Munich Octoberfest: results from the Munich Beer Related Electrocardiogram Workup Study (MunichBREW). Eur Heart J. 2017 Apr 25.

6.   Fan AZ, Russell M, Naimi T, Li Y, Liao Y, et al. (2008) Patterns of alcohol consumption and the metabolic syndrome. J Clin Endocrinol Metab 93: 3833–3838.

9. BRUSHING

Introduction

History tells us that tooth brushing was practiced as far back as 3000 BC, when the ancient Egyptians used crude toothbrushes made from twigs and leaves to clean their teeth. Twigs have also been used by other cultures including the Greeks, Romans, Arabs and Indians to clean teeth. The modern toothbrush consists of a small brush on a handle and is used to clean the teeth with toothpaste – an abrasive gel or paste that helps in removing plaque from teeth. It also suppresses halitosis and may help prevent tooth decay and gum disease by delivering active ingredients such as fluoride. Regular brushing of the teeth also helps prevent periodontal disease. Periodontal disease, a chronic infection of the tissues surrounding the teeth, results in increased inflammation. Inflammation is a major player in the pathogenesis of atherosclerosis. Poor dental hygiene therefore raises the risk of cardiovascular disease. The World Health Organization estimates that 10%-20% of the world population suffer from severe periodontal disease.[1]

Scientific Evidence

- Periodontal disease due to poor oral hygiene initiates a systemic inflammatory response.[2] This inflammatory response is accompanied by an elevation of several inflammatory biomarker levels in the blood, such as C-reactive protein and interleukin-6.[3] Diminished frequency of tooth brushing is also associated with elevated C-reactive protein levels.[4]
- Systemic inflammation may lead to the initiation, progression, and ultimately the thrombotic complications of atherosclerosis.[5] Atherosclerosis gives rise to plaques in the arteries, which harden and eventually narrow the vessel or may be suddenly blocked by the development of a blood clot, cutting off the blood supply to the intended organ. This may cause a heart attack, stroke and even death.[6]
- Periodontitis has been shown to increase the risk of cardiovascular diseases and stroke.[7]

- In a study with follow up data of 15 years and involving 9,760 subjects (First National Health and Nutritional Examination Survey Epidemiologic Follow-up Study), researchers noted that there was a 25% increase in the risk for coronary heart disease in patients with periodontal disease.[8]

- In a longitudinal study, mean bone loss scores and worst probing pocket depth scores per tooth were measured on 1,147 men during the years 1968 to 1971. Researchers found that among people with periodontal bone loss, there was 50% increased risk for coronary heart disease and a 90% increased risk for fatal coronary artery disease.[9]

- In a study involving 4,830 participants, 555 cardiovascular disease events occurred over an average of 8.1 years of follow-up, resulting in 170 deaths. Participants with poor oral hygiene had a 70% increased risk when compared to those with good oral hygiene.[4]

- In a retrospective study, the medical records of 90,143 individuals who had undergone an annual medical checkup were reviewed. Researchers found that a lower frequency of tooth brushing was associated with high prevalence of diabetes mellitus and dyslipidemia – major risk factors for cardiovascular diseases.[10]

Conclusion

The association between poor oral hygiene and the risk of cardiovascular disease is well documented. Regular brushing decreases inflammatory markers in the blood and reduces the risk of premature heart attack and/or cardiovascular death.

Lifestyle Implications

Brush your teeth twice a day and change your toothbrush (soft bristles) every three months. Regular dental flossing can help keep the inter-dental areas free of tarter.

References

1. Petersen PE. The World Oral Health Report 2003: continuous improvement of oral health in the 21st century—the approach of the WHO global oral health programme. Community Dent Oral Epidemiol2003;31(suppl 1):3-23S.
2. D'Aiuto F, Ready D, Tonetti MS. Periodontal disease and C-reactive protein-associated cardiovascular risk. J Periodont Res 2004;39:236-41.

3. Loos BG, Craandijk J, Hoek FJ, Wertheim-van Dillen PM, van der Velden U. Elevation of systemic markers related to cardiovascular diseases in the peripheral blood of periodontitis patients. J Periodontol 2000;71:1528-34.

4. de Oliveira Cesar, Watt Richard, Hamer Mark. Toothbrushing, inflammation, and risk of cardiovascular disease: results from Scottish Health Survey BMJ 2010; 340: c2451.

5. Peter Libby, Paul M. Ridker and Attilio Maseri. Inflammation and Atherosclerosis. Circulation. 2002;105:1135-1143.

6. https://www.nhlbi.nih.gov/health/health-topics/topics/atherosclerosis

7. Persson GR, Persson RE. Cardiovascular disease and periodontitis: an update on the associations and risk. J Clin Periodontol 2008;35:362-79.

8. DeStefano F, Anda RF, Kahn HS, Williamson DF, Russell CM. Dental disease and risk of coronary heart disease and mortality. BMJ 1993;306:688-91.

9. Beck J, Garcia R, Heiss G, Vokonas PS, Offenbacher S. Periodontal disease and cardiovascular disease. J Periodontol 1996;67:1123-37.

10. Kuwabara M, Motoki Y, Ichiura K et al. Association between toothbrushing and risk factors for cardiovascular disease: a large-scale, cross-sectional Japanese study. BMJ Open. 2016 Jan 14;6(1): e009870.

10. BUTTER

Introduction

Butter is used all over the world as a spread on bread, a condiment on cooked vegetables or seafood, and in cooking. It is usually made from cows' milk, but can also be produced from the milk of buffalo, camel, goat, ewe, and mares. It is formed by churning fresh or fermented cream or milk. This process separates the butterfat (the solids) from the buttermilk (the liquid). Butter is high in saturated fats - it is usually 80% fat, 16% water and 3% milk solids. Ghee is purified butter and is more stable in warmer climates. The Hindu sacred book, Bhagavad Gita, dating back to the 2nd century BC, mentions ghee in its text. It has also been mentioned numerous times in the Rigveda, circa 1500–1200 BC. Ghee may be higher in anti-oxidants than regular butter. Butter contains only trace amounts of lactose and is easily tolerated by lactose intolerant people. Besides saturated fat, butter is also a good source of vitamin A. Because of its high concentration of saturated fats, consumption of butter is considered a risk factor for atherosclerosis – which is the main cause of heart attacks and strokes. However, emerging evidence suggests that intake of butter, a diary fat, may be associated with cardiometabolic benefits.

Scientific Evidence

- In 1970, the Seven Countries Study found that populations with elevated serum cholesterol levels and those consuming high levels of saturated fats had high levels of coronary heart disease and thrombotic stroke.[1]
- In 1987, the Henry J. Kaiser Family Foundation, along with twenty-three national associations, launched Project LEAN (Low-Fat Eating for America Now), which encouraged Americans to reduce total fat intake to 30 percent of their diet.[2]
- In 1997, Frank Hu, based on data collected from 80,082 women enrolled in the long-running Nurses' Health Study, confirmed the hypothesis that a higher dietary intake of saturated fat and trans unsaturated fat was associated with an increased risk of coronary disease, whereas a higher intake of monounsaturated and polyunsaturated fats was associated with a reduced risk. Their data

suggested that replacing 5 percent of saturated fat calories with unsaturated fat would reduce the risk of heart disease by 42 percent and replacing only 2 percent of trans-fat calories with unsaturated fat would reduce the risk of heart disease by 53 percent.[3]

- In 2014, a meta-analysis was published that questioned the then current cardiovascular guidelines that encouraged high consumption of polyunsaturated fatty acids and low consumption of total saturated fats.[4]

- A recent systematic review and meta-analysis revealed a relatively small or neutral overall association of butter with mortality, cardiovascular disease, and diabetes. This investigation included a review of data from 9 studies - involving 636,151 participants with 6.5 million person-years of follow-up. There were 28,271 total deaths, 9,783 cases of incident cardiovascular disease, and 23,954 cases of incident diabetes in this population during the period of the study.[5]

- Saturated fats may actually help increase the 'good' high density lipoprotein cholesterol and lower the 'bad' very low-density lipoprotein cholesterol and chylomicron remnants, and lower lipoprotein(a).[6]

Conclusion

Several recent articles have called into question the purported deleterious effects of some high animal fats. Butter is high in saturated diary fat. Recent systematic review and meta-analysis suggests that the relationship between butter and cardiovascular disease and death is probably neutral. Butter can therefore be consumed without concern, provided the daily intake does not lead to over 10 percent of calories coming from saturated fats.[7]

Lifestyle Implications

It is okay to eat butter, in moderation.

References

1. Keys, Ancel, C. Aravanis, H. Blackburn et al. 1980. Seven countries. A multivariate analysis of death and coronary heart disease. Cambridge: Harvard University Press.
2. Project LEAN, AJPH March 1989, Vol. 79, No. 3

3. Frank B. Hu, M.D., Meir J. Stampfer, M.D., et al. Dietary Fat Intake and the Risk of Coronary Heart Disease in Women. N Engl J Med 1997; 337:1491-1499 November 20, 1997.

4. Chowdhury R, Warnakula S, Kunutsor S, et al. Association of dietary, circulating, and supplement fatty acids with coronary risk. Ann Intern Med 2014; 160(6):398-406.

5. Pimpin L, Wu JHY, Haskelberg H, Del Gobbo L, Mozaffarian D. Is Butter Back? A Systematic Review and Meta-Analysis of Butter Consumption and Risk of Cardiovascular Disease, Diabetes, and Total Mortality. Schooling CM, ed. PLoS ONE. 2016;11(6): e0158118.

6. van Schalkwijk DB, Pasman WJ, Hendriks HF, et al. Dietary medium chain fatty acid supplementation leads to reduced VLDL lipolysis and uptake rates in comparison to linoleic acid supplementation. PLoS One. 2014; 9(7): e100376

7. HHS and USDA Release New Dietary Guidelines to Encourage Healthy Eating Patterns to Prevent Chronic Diseases. Available at dietaryguidelines.gov.

11. CALCIUM SUPPLEMENTS

Introduction

Calcium is the fifth most abundant element in the human body. More than 99% of the body stores of calcium reside in the skeleton, not only providing support to the bones but also as a reservoir to maintain proper serum calcium concentrations. The circulating levels of calcium in the body are usually maintained in a constant range of 1.0 to 1.2 mmol/L.[1] Low calcium intake from dietary sources leads to a compensatory loss of calcium from the bones, weakening the skeleton and increasing the risk of subsequent fracture.[2] It is this fear of developing osteoporosis that drives almost 70% of older women to take calcium supplements in the United States. Overall, about 43% of US residents take supplements that contain calcium. Most recent reports suggest that excessive intake of calcium may lead to a higher risk of cardiovascular events, while some have concluded otherwise.

Scientific Evidence

- Calcium helps lower blood pressure. In 2006, a Cochrane review including 13 randomized control trials demonstrated a reduction in systolic blood pressure by 2.5 mm Hg in hypertensive patients, with calcium supplementation.[3]
- A large study, the Women's Health Initiative, reported no adverse effect of calcium and vitamin D (1 g calcium/400 IU vitamin D daily) on cardiovascular end points. This study included 36,282 participants and was a seven year, randomized, placebo controlled trial. However, the data was deemed unreliable due to self-administration of supplements by many participants prior to enrollment.[4]
- In a meta-analysis of five studies with 8,151 participants followed for a median period of 3.6 years and another 11 studies with 11,921 participants followed over a mean duration of 4 years, researchers concluded that calcium supplements result in 31% increased incidence of myocardial infarction, if taken without co-administered vitamin D.[5]
- A subsequent study found that calcium supplements with or without vitamin D modestly increased the risk of cardiovascular events, especially myocardial infarction. This was a seven year,

randomized, placebo controlled trial of calcium and vitamin D (1g calcium and 400 IU vitamin D daily) in 36,282 community dwelling, postmenopausal women.[6]

- In a meta-analysis of 11 prospective observational studies, Larsson and associates found that in those with low dietary calcium intake (<700 mg/d), a 300 mg/d increase in calcium intake was associated with a reduction in stroke risk, whereas a slightly increased risk of stroke was seen in those with high dietary calcium intake ($\geq$700 mg/d).[7]
- A recently published review suggests a significant increase in incident coronary artery calcification with calcium supplementation.[8]

Conclusion

Calcium is an important nutrient for humans. For adults, the recommended daily intake of calcium is 1,000 milligrams up to age 50 in women. That amount increases to 1,200 mg per day for women over 50 years and men older than 70 years.[9] However, data indicates that meeting dietary goals of calcium intake may be cardio-vascular wise healthier if done without supplementation Three daily servings of calcium rich foods can help meet the recommended requirements. Foods rich in calcium include milk, yogurt, cheese, canned oily fish with bones, tofu, calcium-fortified juice, and leafy greens. Those unable to take dairy foods due to lactose intolerance may take a calcium supplement of 500 to 700 mg per day with their health providers consent – higher amounts could be harmful.

Lifestyle Implications

Calcium supplements should be avoided.

References

1. Ross AC, Taylor CL, Yaktine AL, del Valle HB: *Dietary Reference Intakes for Calcium and Vitamin D*. National Academies Press; 2010.
2. Institute of Medicine. Dietary reference intakes for calcium and vitamin D. Washington, DC: Institute of Medicine; 2010. Available from: http://www.iom.edu/Reports/2010/Dietary-Reference-Intakes-for-Calcium-and-Vitamin-D.aspx.
3. Dickinson HO, Nicolson DJ, Cook JV, et al. Calcium supplementation for the management of primary hypertension in adults. *Cochrane Database Syst Rev.* 2006;2:CD004639.

4. Hsia J, Heiss G, Ren H, et al. Women's Health Initiative Investigators. Calcium/vitamin D supplementation and cardiovascular events. Circulation. 2007 Feb 20; 115(7):846-54.

5. Bolland MJ, Avenell A, Baron JA, et al. Effect of calcium supplements on risk of myocardial infarction and cardiovascular events: meta-analysis. *The BMJ*. 2010;341:c3691.

6. Bolland MJ, Grey A, Avenell A, Gamble GD, Reid IR. Calcium supplements with or without vitamin D and risk of cardiovascular events: reanalysis of the Women's Health Initiative limited access dataset and meta-analysis. *The BMJ*. 2011; 342: d2040.

7. Larsson SC, Orsini N, Wolk A. Dietary calcium intake and risk of stroke: a dose-response meta-analysis. Am J Clin Nutr. 2013;97:951–957.

8. Aurel T. Tankeu MD, Valirie Ndip Agbor MD, Jean Jacques Noubiap MD. Calcium supplementation and cardiovascular risk: A rising concern. JCH, 2 May 2017.

9. Institute of Medicine. Dietary Reference Intakes for Calcium and Vitamin D. Washington, DC: National Academies Press; 2011.

12. CARBOHYDRATES

Introduction

Carbohydrates provide about 40% to 60% of the energy needed for the body. However, excess carbohydrates that are not used get converted to and are stored as fat. Carbohydrates are of four types, namely monosaccharides containing a single sugar such as glucose and fructose, disaccharides containing two monosaccharides such as sucrose and lactose, oligosaccharides with short chains, and polysaccharides with long chains such as starch, glycogen (these store energy), cellulose and chitin (these help build structural components). Simple carbohydrates are abundant in foods such as candy, jams, and desserts. Foods such as bread, pasta, potatoes and cereals have high levels of complex carbohydrates. The rate and degree of rise of blood sugar with ingestion of carbohydrates have established the glycemic index (GI). Low GI value carbohydrates are usually digested, absorbed and metabolized slowly and cause a lower and slower rise in blood glucose and insulin levels. This is heart healthy. Foods with low GI (less than 55) include soy products, beans, most fruits and vegetables, milk, pasta, grainy bread, porridge and lentils. Those with medium GI (55 to 70) include corn, white rice, orange juice, honey, and whole-meal bread. Those with high GI (greater than 70) include potatoes, donuts, bagels, cakes, white bread, corn flakes, high fructose corn syrup and short-grain rice. Other factors affecting the cardiovascular system include the fiber and whole grain content of the carbohydrates consumed, as well as the total calories.[1]

Scientific Evidence

- The quality rather than the quantity of carbohydrates appears to be a stronger determinant of future cardiovascular disease. The former includes the fiber content, the glycemic index, amount of processing, and the whole grain content.[2]
- Observational studies have identified post-challenge hyperglycemia as an independent risk factor for cardiovascular disease, suggesting that carbohydrates with a high glycemic index are harmful.[3] A high GI is also associated with a higher prevalence of the metabolic syndrome, as noted in the Framingham Offspring Cohort Study.[4]

- In a study of 2,941 Framingham Offspring Participants, dietary GI was significantly associated with several cardiovascular disease risk factors, including high triacylglycerol concentrations, low high-density lipoprotein cholesterol concentrations and abnormal insulin levels and sensitivity.[5]
- Carbohydrates with high-fiber not only protect against obesity, but also reduce the risk of cardiovascular disease, especially by lowering insulin levels.[6]
- Carbohydrate intake as whole grains also reduces the risk of cardiovascular disease.[1] Whole grains contain endosperm, germ, and bran, while refining removes the germ and bran during the milling process. The germ and bran contain most of the cardioprotective nutrients.
- Excess intake of carbohydrates, especially refined grains, starches, and sugar, lead to long term obesity.[7] Obesity, especially visceral obesity, results in deleterious cardio-metabolic changes and further potentiates the development and progression of cardiovascular diseases.

Conclusion

Carbohydrates eaten in excess will result in obesity – a risk factor for cardiovascular disease. Carbohydrates that are rich in fiber, whole grains, require little processing, and have a low glycemic index are cardioprotective. Following a low glycemic index diet also helps shed weight and reduce the risk of developing diabetes mellitus and age-related macular degeneration. It is heart healthy to avoid processed foods that have sugar added to improve their taste – such as sugar-sweetened beverages, fruit flavored drinks, desserts, candy and ready to eat cereals.

Lifestyle Implications

Low glycemic index carbohydrates are cardio-protective.

References

1. Aune Dagfinn, Keum NaNa, Giovannucci Edward, Fadnes Lars T, Boffetta Paolo, Greenwood Darren C et al. Whole grain consumption and risk of cardiovascular disease, cancer, and all cause and cause specific mortality: systematic review and dose-response meta-analysis of prospective studies BMJ 2016; 353 :i2716.

2.   Mozaffarian D, Appel LJ, Van Horn L. Components of a cardioprotective diet: new insights. Circulation. 2011;123:2870–2891.

3.   de Vegt F, Dekker JM, Ruhé HG, et al. Hyperglycaemia is associated with all-cause and cardiovascular mortality in the Hoorn population: the Hoorn Study. Diabetologia. 1999 Aug; 42(8):926-31.

4.   McKeown NM, Meigs JB, Liu S, Saltzman E, Wilson PW, Jacques PF. Carbohydrate nutrition, insulin resistance, and the prevalence of the metabolic syndrome in the Framingham Offspring Cohort. Diabetes Care. 2004;27:538–546.

5.   McKeown NM, Meigs JB, Liu S, et al. Dietary Carbohydrates and Cardiovascular Disease Risk Factors in the Framingham Offspring Cohort. Journal of the American College of Nutrition. 2009;28(2):150-158.

6.   Ludwig DS, Pereira MA, Kroenke CH, Hilner JE, Van Horn L, Slattery ML, Jacobs, Jr DR. Dietary Fiber, Weight Gain, and Cardiovascular Disease Risk Factors in Young Adults. JAMA. 1999;282(16):1539–1546.

7.   Smith JD, Hou T, Ludwig DS, et al. Changes in intake of protein foods, carbohydrate amount and quality, and long-term weight change: results from 3 prospective cohorts. Am J Clin Nutr. 2015;101:1216–1224.

13. CHEESE

Introduction

Cheese is a popular food worldwide. It is estimated that in 2014, cheese production from cow milk was 18.7 million tons, globally. Its production and consumption predates recorded human history. Archaeological evidence of cheese making (strainers with milk fat molecules) has been found in Poland, dating back to 5,500 BCE. Cheese is formed by the coagulation of the milk protein casein. Commonly used milk for cheese production comes from cows, buffalo, goats, or sheep. Cheese is rich in fat, protein, calcium, and phosphorus. The International Dairy Federation recognizes 500 different varieties of cheese. Because of its fat content, questions have been raised about its effects on the cardiovascular system.

Scientific Evidence

- Blood pressure may be beneficially influenced by low-fat dairy products.[1]
- A meta-analysis of 29 cohort studies, with 938,465 participants and 93,158 deaths, (28,419 from coronary heart disease and 25,416 from cardiovascular diseases) revealed no associations between total (high-fat/low-fat) dairy consumption and cardiovascular mortality.[2]
- In a meta-analysis of thirty-one cohort studies, researchers concluded that dairy consumption may be associated with reduced risks of cardiovascular disease.[3]
- In another meta-analysis of 22 studies, investigators found an inverse association between dairy consumption and the overall risk of cardiovascular disease. Interestingly, cheese consumption was associated with a significant (26%) reduction in the risk of coronary heart disease.[4]
- Dairy products are rich in minerals (calcium, potassium, and magnesium), protein (casein and whey), and vitamins (riboflavin and vitamin B-12) - these may exert beneficial effects on cardiovascular health.

Conclusion

Cheese is widely consumed all over the world. Because it is rich in fat, concern has been raised about its ability to increase cardiovascular disease. However, several studies, including major meta-analysis studies, demonstrate neutral or slightly beneficial associations between intake of cheese and cardiovascular diseases, and all-cause mortality. Cheese may be eaten without worry, but as with most foods, in moderation. Some cheeses are high in sodium, and may cause a worsening of high blood pressure and heart failure.

Lifestyle Implications

Moderate cheese intake appears safe for the heart. Avoid cheese with high saturated fat and high sodium levels.

References

1. Toledo E, Delgado-Rodriguez M, Estruch R, et al. Low-fat dairy products and blood pressure: follow-up of 2290 older persons at high cardiovascular risk participating in the PREDIMED study. Br J Nutr 2009;101:59–67.
2. Soedamah-Muthu SS, Ding EL, Al-Delaimy WK, Hu FB, Engberink MF, Willett WC, Geleijnse JM. Milk and dairy consumption and incidence of cardiovascular diseases and all-cause mortality: dose-response meta-analysis of prospective cohort studies. Am J Clin Nutr. 2011;93:158–171.
3. Alexander DD, Bylsma LC, Vargas AJ, Cohen SS, Doucette A, Mohamed M, Irvin SR, Miller PE, Watson H, Fryzek JP. Dairy consumption and CVD: a systematic review and meta-analysis. Br J Nutr. 2016 Feb 28;115(4):737-50.
4. Qin LQ, Xu JY, Han SF, Zhang ZL, Zhao YY, Szeto IM. Dairy consumption and risk of cardiovascular disease: an updated meta-analysis of prospective cohort studies. Asia Pac J Clin Nutr. 2015;24(1):90-100.

14. CHILDREN

Introduction

A human being below the age of 18 years is considered a child. Biologically a child is anyone between birth and the onset of puberty. There are several emotional and social benefits to parents from having children. However, children are expensive to raise. The Department of Agriculture has estimated that a middle-income, married couple with two children will spend $233,610 to raise a child born in 2015 (through age 17). College expenses may be more. Children can be a factor influencing the risk for cardiovascular disease, in the parents. Recent scientific studies have recognized that having no children or having more than two children is stressful to the cardiovascular system.

Scientific Evidence

- Many studies have found a positive association between parity and mortality from cardiovascular and cerebrovascular diseases.[1,2]
- In a large study of 4,286 women and 4,252 men aged 60 to 79 years from 24 British towns, researchers noted that having more than 2 children was associated with increased parental obesity and increased coronary artery disease in both parents. For those with at least 2 children, the risk of coronary artery disease increased by 30% in women and 12% in men for each additional child.[3] Pregnancy and having children in women was also associated with adverse lipid profiles and diabetes.
- In another British study of 2,977 individuals (51% women), investigators found no clear relationship between the number of children and coronary heart disease risk factors at age 53 years. They did record an increased tendency towards obesity and higher HbA1c (both risk factors for coronary artery disease) in both men and women with increasing number of children.[4]
- In the NIH-AARP Diet and Health Study, 137,903 men (aged 50–71), without prior cardiovascular disease, were monitored for an average of 10.2 years. A review of the data revealed that when compared to fathers, after adjusting for sociodemographic and lifestyle factors, childless men had a 17% increased risk of death from cardiovascular disease.[5]

- In another study of 12,055 women with children, followed during the years 1966-2001, researchers found that high parity was associated with an increased risk of mortality from vascular complications, especially hemorrhagic stroke.[6] The increased risk of stroke in women with many pregnancies when compared to women who were nulligravida, has been reported before.[7]

- Another study enrolled 39,876 women aged ≥45 years without cardiovascular disease or any major illness. Researchers found that atrial fibrillation was more common in women with multiple pregnancies when compared with nulliparous women.[8]

- In a large study of 0.5 million individuals aged 30–79 years, without prior cardiovascular disease and followed for 7 years, 24,432 incident cases of coronary heart disease and 35,736 of stroke were recorded. Compared with childless women and men, those with children had an increased risk of coronary heart disease.[9]

Conclusion

Increased parity is associated with a higher risk of cardiovascular disease in both men and women. Besides the metabolic changes associated with pregnancy in women, having more children may also increase the economic and social stress on the parents.

Lifestyle Implications

One or two children appear to be heart protective for the parents. Less or more may be bad for the heart.

References

1. Beral V. Long term effects of childbearing on health. J Epidemiol Commun Health 1985, 39343–346.

2. Hinkula M, Kauppila A, Näyhä S. et al Cause-specific mortality of grand multiparous women in Finland. Am J Epidemiol 20054367–373.

3. A. Lawlor, MPH, MBchB; Jonathan R. Emberson, et al. Is the Association Between Parity and Coronary HeartDisease Due to Biological Effects of Pregnancy or AdverseLifestyle Risk Factors Associated With Child-Rearing? Findings From the British Women's Heart and Health Study and theBritish Regional Heart Study. Circulation. 2003;107:1260-1264.

4. R Hardy, DA Lawlor, S Black, MEJ Wadsworth, D Kuh. Number of children and coronary heart disease risk factors in men and women from a British birth cohort. BJOG 16 May 2007.

5. Eisenberg ML, Park Y, Hollenbeck AR, Lipshultz LI, Schatzkin A, Pletcher MJ. Fatherhood and the risk of cardiovascular mortality in the NIH-AARP Diet and Health Study. Human Reproduction (Oxford, England). 2011;26(12):3479-3485.

6. Koski-Rahikkala H, Pouta A, Pietiläinen K, Hartikainen A. Does parity affect mortality among parous women? Journal of Epidemiology and Community Health. 2006;60(11):968-973.

7. Qureshi AI, Giles WH, Croft JB, Stern BJ. Number of pregnancies and risk for stroke and stroke subtypes. Arch Neurol. 1997 Feb;54(2):203-6.

8. Jorge A. Wong, Kathryn M. Rexrode, Roopinder K. Sandhu, David Conen and Christine M. Albert. Number of Pregnancies and Atrial Fibrillation Risk. Circulation. 2017;135:622-624.

9. Sanne AE, Peters, Ling Yang, Yu Guo, et al. Parenthood and the risk of cardiovascular diseases among 0.5 million men and women: findings from the China Kadoorie Biobank. International Journal of Epidemiology, Volume 46, Issue 1, 1 February 2017, Pages 180–189.

15. CHOCOLATE

Introduction

Cocoa products have been enjoyed by humans for centuries. Chocolate is made from cocoa (cacao) and has a good taste. Theobroma caca, the source of cacoa, grows in the subtropical areas of the world. Although it grows widely from the southeastern Mexico to the Amazon basin, two thirds of the world's production comes from four West African countries - the Ivory Coast, Ghana, Nigeria and Cameroon. The medicinal value of cocao beans was recognized by American researchers when they noticed that residents of the island Kuna in South America drank large amounts of home-prepared cocoa, rich in flavonoids, and remained hypertension free. The Kuna on the mainland, however, consumed commercial cocoa devoid of flavonoids, and developed hypertension and cardiovascular diseases.[1] Cocoa is rich in flavonoids which protect against cardiovascular diseases through their antioxidant, antiplatelet, and anti-inflammatory effects.

Scientific Evidence

- In a meta-analysis, higher levels of chocolate consumption were associated with a reduction of cardiovascular disease by 37%, diabetes by 31% and stroke by 29%.[2]

- Cocoa is beneficial in preventing high blood pressure. Its consumption is inversely related to blood pressure.[3,4] The benefits from its consumption are noted in both healthy and in hypertensive populations.

- Cocoa consumption is also lipid beneficial. A consumption of 100 gm of flavonoid rich chocolate for over 2 weeks was associated with a 12% reduction in total and low-density lipoprotein cholesterol levels in patients.[5] Cocoa also inhibits oxidative damage of the low-density lipoprotein cholesterol – preventing the formation of foam cells and the deadly atherosclerosis. There is an increase in the beneficial high-density lipoprotein cholesterol concentration.

- In a large trial involving 37,103 men and monitored for 10.2 years, there were 1,995 incident stroke cases (1,511 cerebral infarctions, 321 hemorrhagic strokes, and 163 unspecified strokes). Review of this data showed an overall 19% decrease in the risk for stroke for the highest consumers of chocolate - male and female - compared with those who consumed the least.[6]

- Cocoa consumption is also associated with a reduction in cardiovascular and all-cause mortality.[3]

- Chocolate intake may also improve insulin sensitivity.[7] In one meta-analysis, higher levels of chocolate consumption were associated with a reduction of diabetes by about 31%.[2] Diabetes mellitus is a major risk factor for cardiovascular diseases.

- These benefits appear due to flavanols in cocoa – they increase nitric oxide bioavailability, protect the vascular endothelium, and decrease cardiovascular disease risk factors.

Conclusion

Epidemiological and scientific studies demonstrate that dark chocolate from cocoa beans is cardioprotective. Chocolate is made by fermenting, roasting and grounding the bitter raw cocao beans and then separating them into cocoa powder and cocoa butter. Dark chocolate has less milk and is produced by adding fat and sugar to cocoa. Unsweetened, dark chocolate contains up to 75% cocoa solids compared with only 20% found in milk chocolate. White chocolate is not made from cocoa beans, but from cocoa butter and is almost devoid of flavonoids. It is estimated that consuming 100 grams of dark chocolate with at least 60-70% cocoa, several times a week, would prevent 70 non-fatal cardiovascular events and 15 cardiovascular deaths per 10.000 population treated over 10 years.[9]

Lifestyle Implications

Chocoholics should continue to enjoy dark chocolate – and will enjoy several health benefits.

References

1. Fisher ND, Hollenberg NK. Flavanols for cardiovascular health: the science behind the sweetness. J Hypertens, 2005, 23(8), 1453-9.
2. Adriana Buitrago-Lopez, Jean Sanderson, Laura Johnson, et al. Chocolate Consumption and Cardiometabolic Disorders. Systematic Review and MetaAnalysis. British Medical Journal, 2011.
3. Buijsse B, Feskens EJ, Kok FJ, Kromhout D. Cocoa intake, blood pressure, and cardiovascular mortality: the Zutphen Elderly Study. Arch Intern Med. 2006;166:411-417.

4.   Buijsse B, Weikert C, Drogan D, Bergmann M, Boeing H. Chocolate consumption in relation to blood pressure and risk of cardiovascular disease in German adults. Eur Heart J 2010, 31, 1616–1623.

5.   Grassi D, Necozione S, Lippi C, et al. Cocoa reduces blood pressure and insulin resistance and improves endothelium-dependent vasodilation in hypertensives. Hypertension. 2005, 46, 398–405.

6.   Susanna C. Larsson, PhD, Jarmo Virtamo, MD and Alicja Wolk, DMSc Chocolate consumption and risk of stroke. A prospective cohort of men and meta-analysis. Neurology. 2012, 79, 1223-1229.

7.   Grassi D, Desideri G, Necozione S, Lippi C, Casale R, Properzi G, Blumberg JB, Ferri C. Blood pressure is reduced and insulin sensitivity increased in glucoseintolerant, hypertensive subjects after 15 days of consuming high-polyphenol dark chocolate. J Nutr 2008, 138, 1671–1676.

8.   Ella Zomer, Alice Owen, Dianna J Magliano, Danny Liew, Christopher M Reid. The Effectiveness and Cost Effectiveness of Dark Chocolate Consumption as Prevention Therapy in People at High Risk of Cardiovascular Disease. British Medical Journal, 2012.

16. CHOLESTEROL

Introduction

Cholesterol is necessary for proper functioning of the human body. Almost 30% of the cell membranes are made up of cholesterol, which helps in maintaining cell integrity and its proper functioning. Cholesterol is also involved in intracellular transport, cell signaling and nerve conduction. It is also a precursor for the synthesis of vitamin D and all steroid and sex hormones. Cholesterol is present in all animal based foods, including cheese, egg yolks, beef, pork, poultry, fish, and shrimp. Infants get their cholesterol from human milk. Cholesterol is not manufactured by plants and is not found in plant food. It is also produced in the liver, the intestines, adrenal glands, and reproductive organs of humans. It is carried in the blood within lipoproteins. The blood contains several lipoproteins, such as chylomicrons, very-low-density lipoproteins, intermediate-density lipoproteins, low-density lipoproteins, and high-density lipoproteins. The low-density lipoprotein is the major cholesterol carrier, and this cholesterol is commonly known as the 'bad' cholesterol. When oxidized and swallowed by macrophages, foam cells are formed, which are instrumental in the formation of the atherosclerotic plaque. High-density lipoprotein carries the 'good' cholesterol, and transports the cholesterol back to the liver, for excretion or other purposes.

Scientific Evidence

- A strong graded association between serum cholesterol and coronary heart disease has been reported by many studies. The higher the low-density lipoprotein cholesterol, the greater the risk, while, the higher the high density lipoprotein cholesterol, the lower the risk.[1]

- Ratios of total cholesterol/ high-density lipoprotein cholesterol and low-density lipoprotein cholesterol / high-density lipoprotein cholesterol are also helpful in predicting future coronary heart disease.[2] In a major study, the Physicians' Health Study, a 1-unit increase in the low-density lipoprotein cholesterol / high-density lipoprotein cholesterol ratio resulted in a 53% increase in the risk of myocardial infarction.[3]

- Treatment with statins significantly reduces the risk for coronary artery morbidity and mortality events - by almost 34%.[4]

- High cholesterol, especially low-density lipoprotein cholesterol, can also be improved by weight loss and several heart healthy diets recommended by different associations.

- Although dietary intake of cholesterol increases total cholesterol and low-density lipoprotein cholesterol levels,[5] a detrimental effect from such a diet is mostly seen in diabetics.[6]

- The role of dietary cholesterol in increasing the risk of heart disease in healthy individuals has not been well established.[7]

Conclusion

The role and association of high serum low-density lipoprotein cholesterol levels and low high-density lipoprotein cholesterol levels and the increased risk of coronary artery disease, both fatal and nonfatal, is well established. Diabetics and those with coronary artery disease or significant risk factors including abnormal cholesterol levels, should limit their consumption of saturated fats, trans-fatty acids and try to achieve a normal body weight. Regular exercise may help increase high-density lipoprotein cholesterol levels. In patients at a high risk for coronary heart disease, it is recommended that the desirable goal for serum low density lipoprotein cholesterol level be <70 mg/dl and that high-density lipoprotein cholesterol be above 60 mg/dl.

Lifestyle Implications

Although dietary intake of cholesterol may not influence coronary artery disease in healthy people, it is wise to monitor the cholesterol levels and keep them within the recommended range. Cholesterol testing should be done every 4–6 years in adults.

References

1. Wilson PW, D'Agostino RB, Levy D, Belanger AM, Silbershatz H, Kannel WB. (1998) Prediction of coronary heart disease using risk factor categories. Circulation; 97(18):1837-47.

2. NIH Consensus Development Panel on Triglyceride, High-Density Lipoprotein, and Coronary Heart Disease. NIH Consensus Conference: Triglyceride, High-Density Lipoprotein, and Coronary Heart Disease. JAMA. 1993;269:505-510.

3. Stampfer MJ, Sacks FM, Salvini S, et al. A prospective study of cholesterol apolipoproteins and the risk of myocardial infarction. N Engl J Med. 1991;325:373-381.

4. 4S Study Group. Randomised trial of cholesterol lowering in 4444 patients with coronary heart disease: the Scandinavian Simvastatin Survival Study (4S). Lancet. 1994;344:1383–1389.

5. Institute of Medicine Dietary reference intakes for energy, carbohydrate, fiber, fat, fatty acids, cholesterol, protein, and amino acids. Washington, DC: National Academies Press; 2002.

6. U.S. Department of Agriculture and U.S. Department of Health and Human Services Dietary guidelines for Americans 2010. 7th ed. Washington, DC: U.S. Government Printing Office, 2010.

7. Kanter MM, Kris-Etherton PM, Fernandez ML, et al. Exploring the Factors That Affect Blood Cholesterol and Heart Disease Risk: Is Dietary Cholesterol as Bad for You as History Leads Us to Believe? Advan in Nutrition. 2012;3(5):711-717.

17. COFFEE

Introduction

Coffee is a popular beverage, having the proud distinction of being the world's second most popular drink, after water. It is usually served as a hot drink, and is made from the seeds of the coffee plant (*Coffea Arabica* and *Coffea Robusta*). Almost 2.5 billion cups (30 ml/cup) of coffee are consumed per day, worldwide. Coffee is a complex chemical mixture with hundreds of compounds including beneficial antioxidants such as caffeine and polyphenols and, minerals such as potassium and magnesium.[1] Coffee reduces inflammation and this may be the underlying mechanism behind many of its positive effects.[2] Benefits of drinking coffee include reduction in the risk of developing diabetes mellitus, cancer, liver diseases and cardiovascular diseases. Mortality from all causes also improves with coffee ingestion.

Scientific Evidence

- Moderate coffee intake was associated with a lower risk for coronary heart disease in a population followed for 10 years.[3]
- In a major study from Japan, 37,742 participants (18,287 men and 19,455 women) aged 40–64 years, without a history of cancer, myocardial infarction, or stroke, were followed for 10.3 years. The study group found that coffee consumption led to a decreased mortality from all causes, and especially from coronary heart disease in women.[4]
- In a recent meta-analysis of thirty-six studies which included 1,279,804 participants and 36,352 cardiovascular disease cases, researchers concluded that moderate coffee consumption had an inverse relationship with cardiovascular disease risk. Consumption of 3–5 cups/day of coffee was associated with the lowest cardiovascular disease risk.[5]
- In a meta-analysis of 9 cohort studies, coffee consumption of 4 cups or more per day resulted in a 17% reduction in the incidence of stroke.[6]
- A meta-analysis of 9 cohort studies of coffee consumption and risk of type 2 diabetes, including 193.473 participants and 8,394 incident cases of type 2 diabetes, higher habitual coffee intake was

associated with a substantial decreased risk of developing type 2 diabetes.[7] Diabetes mellitus is a major risk factor for cardiovascular diseases. Coffee increases insulin sensitivity.

- In another analysis, involving more than 400,000 participants and 52,000 deaths, there was a dose dependent inverse association between coffee consumption and mortality from all causes. Men who drank 6 or more cups of coffee per day had a 10% lower risk of death, compared to men who did not drink coffee. A 15% lower risk was noted in women in the coffee drinker category.[8]

- In a recently published prospective study involving 3,195,484 person-years of monitoring, there were 58,397 deaths during an average follow up of 16.2 years. Compared with drinking no coffee, coffee consumption was associated with lower total death in African Americans, Japanese Americans, Latinos, and whites.[9]

Conclusion

Coffee is a popular drink and contains several health beneficial compounds. Regular consumption has been associated with a reduced risk for developing cardiovascular diseases and diabetes mellitus. A beneficial effect is also seen on some liver ailments, especially liver cancer. People who habitually drink coffee also live longer. Drinking three to five cups of coffee (8 oz. each cup) per day can be part of a healthy diet, according to the Dietary Guidelines for Americans.[10]

Lifestyle Implications

Drinking coffee is good for cardiovascular protection.

References

1   Gómez-Ruiz JA, Leake DS, Ames JM. In vitro antioxidant activity of coffee compounds and their metabolites. J Agric Food Chem. 2007;55:6962–9.

2   Andersen LF, Jacobs DR, Jr, Carlsen MH, Blomhoff R. Consumption of coffee is associated with reduced risk of death attributed to inflammatory and cardiovascular diseases in the Iowa Women's Health Study. Am J Clin Nutr. 2006;83:1039–46.

3   Wu JN, Ho SC, Zhou C, et al. Coffee consumption and risk of coronary heart diseases: a meta-analysis of 21 prospective cohort studies. Int J Cardiol. 2009, 137, 216-225.

4   Sugiyama K, Kuriyama S, Akhter M, et al. Coffee consumption and mortality due to all causes, cardiovascular disease, and cancer in Japanese women. The Journal of nutrition. 2010;140:1007–1013.

5   Ding M, Bhupathiraju SN, Satija A, et al. Long-Term Coffee Consumption and Risk of Cardiovascular Disease: A Systematic Review and a Dose-Response Meta-Analysis of Prospective Cohort Studies. Circulation. 2014;129(6):643-659.

6   Kim B, Nam Y, Kim J, Choi H, Won C. Coffee Consumption and Stroke Risk: A Meta-analysis of Epidemiologic Studies. Korean Journal of Family Medicine. 2012;33(6):356-365.

7   van Dam RM, Hu FB. Coffee consumption and risk of type 2 diabetes: A systematic review. JAMA. 2005;294:97–104.

8   Freedman ND, Park Y, Abnet CC, Hollenbeck AR, Sinha R. Association of Coffee Drinking with Total and Cause-Specific Mortality. The New England journal of medicine. 2012;366(20):1891-1904.

9   Park S, Freedman ND, Haiman CA, et al. Association of Coffee Consumption With Total and Cause-Specific Mortality Among Nonwhite Populations. Ann Intern Med. [Epub ahead of print 11 July 2017] doi: 10.7326/M16-2472

10 http://health.gov/dietaryguidelines/

18. DANCING

Introduction

Dancing is an enjoyable social activity. Moving to music in a rhythmic way and following a set sequence of steps, is a ubiquitous human social pastime. Throughout history, different human societies developed their own dancing style. Dancing has been depicted on stone and pottery in Greece and Egypt, several thousand years ago. Many dancing rituals were used in ancient times, often to appease higher forces and to remove evil spirits –the main benefit however was always a better health. Today, dancing is done for many reasons - as a healthy exercise, as an entertainment, to express emotions, as a social activity and as an expression of love to somebody or even as a prayer to the Supreme. Competitive dancing has also become common. Health benefits attributed to regular dancing include increased muscular and bone strength, enhanced fitness, better coordination, agility and flexibility, and improved balance. Psychologically there is increased physical confidence, and, greater psychological self-confidence and self-esteem. Social skills are improved.[1] There is also an improvement in the cardiopulmonary health.

Scientific Evidence

- The 2008 Physical Activity Guidelines for Americans recommended a minimum of 75 minutes of vigorous-intensity or 150 minutes of moderate-intensity aerobic activity per week, for health benefits. They suggested that additional benefits can be obtained by doing more than double this amount.[2]
- Lower doses of exercise are also beneficial. In a study involving 122,417 participants, with a mean follow-up of 9.8 ± 2.7 years and 18,122 reported deaths (14.8%), researchers found that a low dose of moderate-to-vigorous-intensity physical activity bestowed a 22% reduction in mortality risk.[3]
- Dance movement therapy improves several cardiovascular parameters and the estimated maximum oxygen consumption in hypertensive patients. These changes translate into a reduction in major cardiovascular events in the future.[4]

- A meta-analysis of four studies showed a positive effect of dance therapy on exercise capacity and blood pressure in hypertensive patients.[5]
- Dancing has a positive effect on psychological well-being, life satisfaction and depression.[6] Depression is negatively associated with cardiovascular diseases.
- A cohort study of 11 independent population surveys in the United Kingdom from 1995 to 2007, with 48,390 adults aged ≥40 years and free of cardiovascular disease at baseline was done by Merom and associates. During the 444,045 person-years of follow-up, 1,714 cardiovascular deaths were documented. Moderate-intensity dancing was associated with an almost 50% reduced risk for cardiovascular disease mortality – better than that seen with walking. The authors postulated that the association between dance and cardiovascular disease mortality may be explained by the high-intensity bouts of exercise during dancing, the lifelong adherence to this activity, and the many psychosocial benefits associated with it.[7]

Conclusion

Dancing (all forms) is a ubiquitous human activity. It positively modulates the health of individuals, whether healthy or burdened with physical and mental ailments. Its benefits in reducing cardiovascular deaths is well documented. Dancing is a good physical, emotional and social activity for humans.

Lifestyle Implications

Enjoy dancing. It is good for your heart.

References

1. https://www.betterhealth.vic.gov.au/health/healthyliving/dance-health-benefits
2. Physical Activity Guidelines Advisory Committee. Physical Activity Guidelines Advisory Committee Report, 2008. Washington, D.C: U.S. Department of Health and Human Services; 2008.
3. Hupin D, Roche F, Gremeaux V, Chatard JC. Even a low-dose of moderate-to-vigorous physical activity reduces mortality by 22% in adults aged ≥60 years: a systematic review and meta-analysis. Br J Sports Med. 2015 Oct;49(19):1262-7.
4. Aweto HA, Owoeye OB, Akinbo SR, Onabajo AA. Effects of dance movement therapy on selected cardiovascular parameters and estimated

maximum oxygen consumption in hypertensive patients. Nig Q J Hosp Med. 2012 Apr-Jun; 22(2):125-9.

5. Lino Sergio Rocha, Mansueto Gomes Neto, Mayra Alves Soares do Amaral et al. Effect of dance therapy on blood pressure and exercise capacity of individuals with hypertension: A systematic review and meta-analysis. International Journal of Cardiology. October 1, 2016 Volume 220, Pages 553–557

6. Konstantinidou, M., Harahousou, Y., & Kambitsis, Ch. (2000). Dance movement therapy effects on life satisfaction of elderly people. In Proceedings of the 6th World Leisure Congress (pp. 207), Bilbao.

7. Merom D, Ding D, Stamatakis E. Dancing Participation and Cardiovascular Disease Mortality: A Pooled Analysis of 11 Population-Based British Cohorts. Am J Prev Med. 2016 Jun;50(6):756-760.

19. DEPRESSION

Introduction

Major depression is a common mental disorder.[1] It carries with it the heaviest burden of disability among mental and behavioral disorders.[2] Its prevalence remains high in people of low socioeconomic status and in those with low education or with a rural background. It is more common in those who are unmarried, separated, or divorced and those without intact families. Depression is associated with increased absenteeism from work and reduced productivity. Other negative consequences often associated with major depression include disruption of family life, alcohol, drug and smoking addictions, and sexual dysfunction. Crime and suicidal behaviors are also common in depressed patients. Patients with major depression also experience accelerated aging, premature mortality, and overall reduced life expectancy. Major depression also has a high rate of co-morbidity and increases the risk of developing or worsening cardiovascular diseases.[3] Treatment of depression is often difficult, despite the availability of many pharmacological and behavioral therapies.

Scientific Evidence

- Many studies have reported a higher incidence of hypertension in patients with depression.[4]
- Depression is associated with a higher risk of incident coronary heart disease. [5]
- Depressed patients also exhibit a higher risk of stroke.[6]
- Patients with established cardiovascular disease fare poorly if there is comorbid depression. It is estimated that one in five patients with coronary artery disease or heart failure and one in three patients with stroke, is depressed.[7-9]
- Depression complicating cardiovascular disease results in an increased risk for recurrent cardiovascular events and an increased cardiovascular mortality.[10-12]
- It is unclear whether treatment of depression with conventional antidepressant therapies such as cognitive behavioral therapy, medications, or combination therapy will decrease cardiovascular events.

- Depression has been shown to increase inflammation, cause autonomic nervous system dysfunction and impair coronary flow. Several other causal mechanisms have also been implicated.

Conclusion

Depression is not only a significant risk factor for the development of coronary artery disease and stroke but is often brought upon by the development of the cardiovascular disease. Its presence portends a poor prognosis. There are many ways to avoid depression. These include staying physically active, being optimistic, socializing, meditation and yoga, getting enough sleep, getting a pet etc.

Lifestyle Implications

Depression damages your heart. Please get help if you are depressed.

References

1. Kessler R.C.and Bromet E.J. The epidemiology of depression across cultures. Annu Rev Public Health. 2013; 34: 119–138.
2. WHO, 2010: http://www.nimh.nih.gov/health/statistics/prevalence/major-depression-among-adults.shtml
3. Saran RK, Puri A, Agarwal M. Depression and the heart. Indian Heart Journal. 2012;64(4):397-401.
4. Meng L, Chen D, Yang Y, Zheng Y, Hui R. Depression increases the risk of hypertension incidence: a meta-analysis of prospective cohort studies. J Hypertens. 2012 May; 30(5):842-51.
5. Nicholson A, Kuper H, Hemingway H. Depression as an aetiologic and prognostic factor in coronary heart disease: a meta-analysis of 6362 events among 146 538 participants in 54 observational studies. Eur Heart J. 2006 Dec; 27(23):2763-74.
6. Pan A, Sun Q, Okereke OI, Rexrode KM, Hu FB. Depression and risk of stroke morbidity and mortality: a meta-analysis and systematic review. JAMA. 2011 Sep 21; 306(11):1241-9.
7. Lane D, Carroll D, Ring C, Beevers DG, Lip GY. The prevalence and persistence of depression and anxiety following myocardial infarction. Br J Health Psychol 2002; 7:11–21.
8. Rutledge T, Reis VA, Linke SE, Greenberg BH, Mills PJ. Depression in heart failure a meta-analytic review of prevalence, intervention effects, and associations with clinical outcomes. J Am Coll Cardiol2006; 48:1527–1537.

9. Hackett ML, Yapa C, Parag V, Anderson CS. Frequency of depression after stroke: a systematic review of observational studies. Stroke. 2005; 36:1330–1340.

10. Nicholson A, Kuper H, Hemingway H. Depression as an aetiologic and prognostic factor in coronary heart disease: a meta-analysis of 6362 events among 146 538 participants in 54 observational studies. Eur Heart J 2006; 27:2763–2774.

11. Bartoli F, Lillia N, Lax A, Crocamo C, Mantero V, Carrà G, Agostoni E, Clerici M. Depression after stroke and risk of mortality: a systematic review and meta-analysis. Stroke Res Treat 2013; 2013:862978

12. Jiang W, Alexander J, Christopher E, Kuchibhatla M, Gaulden LH, Cuffe MS, Blazing MA, Davenport C, Califf RM, Krishnan RR, O'Connor CM. Relationship of depression to increased risk of mortality and rehospitalization in patients with congestive heart failure. Arch Intern Med 2001; 161:1849–1856.

20. DIABETES

Introduction

Type 2 diabetes is a leading public health issue globally. Its worldwide prevalence is expected to continue rising - to an estimated 552 million diabetic adults by 2030.[1] It is also a leading cause of death and disability.[2] Diabetes is diagnosed if the fasting blood sugar level is126 mg/dL or higher on two separate tests. A random blood sugar level of 200 mg/dL or higher also suggests diabetes. A glycated hemoglobin (A1C) measurement with a level of 6.5 percent or higher on two separate occasions also indicates diabetes. Another test used to diagnose this disease is the glucose tolerance test. After an overnight fast, the fasting blood sugar level is measured. After drinking a sugary liquid, blood sugar levels are tested periodically for the next several hours. A reading of more than 200 mg/dL after two hours indicates diabetes. Diabetes is associated with an increased risk for several diseases, particularly, cardiovascular disease. The latter is responsible for almost 65% of the deaths in these patients.[3]

Scientific Evidence

- A plethora of epidemiological and pathological data has confirmed the aggressive progression of coronary heart disease in patients with diabetes. Diabetes is now considered as an independent major risk factor for cardiovascular diseases, in both men and women.[4]
- Cardiovascular diseases are responsible for almost 65% of deaths in patients with diabetes.[5]
- Diabetic patients with cardiovascular diseases face a worse prognosis for survival than do cardiovascular disease patients without diabetes.[6]
- Patients with both diabetes and ischemic heart disease are at an increased risk to develop heart failure due to diabetic cardiomyopathy.[7]
- Mortality from stroke is increased almost 3-fold in patients with diabetes when compared with those without diabetes.[8]
- The etiology behind the accelerated cardiovascular disease with poorer prognosis in diabetes is multifactorial.

Conclusion

Diabetes is a dangerous disease. According to the American Diabetes Association, everyone aged 45 and over should be tested for diabetes, and if the results are normal, re-tested every three years. Earlier testing is recommended if a person has the following diabetes risk factors: a parent or sibling with diabetes. being overweight (BMI higher than 25), belonging to a high-risk ethnic population (African American, Hispanic American, Native American, Asian American or Pacific Islander), having gestational diabetes or giving birth to a baby weighing over 9 pounds, abnormal lipid profile with high-density lipoprotein cholesterol levels of 35 mg/dl or less, and/or triglyceride levels of 250 mg/dl or above, being hypertensive, or having polycystic ovarian syndrome. Prevention of type 2 diabetes is primarily achieved by adhering to a proper nutrition, (preferential intake of fruits, vegetables, reduced saturated fat, and low-fat dairy products) weight management (controlled caloric intake, pharmacologic intervention and bariatric surgery) and being physical active (regular aerobic activity 3 to 5 days/week). Supplementation with some antioxidant vitamins, B vitamins, or specific fatty acids (e.g., omega-3 fatty acids) may help in reducing the risk of cardiovascular diseases in these patients. The role of low dose aspirin as a preventive modality is reasonable in adults with diabetes mellitus at intermediate risk (a 10-year cardiovascular risk of 5–10%)

Lifestyle Implications

You can prevent or delay the onset, and/or reduce the severity and progression of diabetes, by following a prudent diet, maintaining a normal BMI, and participating in regular physical exercise.

References

1. Lam D. W., LeRoith D. The worldwide diabetes epidemic. Current Opinion in Endocrinology, Diabetes and Obesity. 2012;19(2):93–96.
2. Bhutani J, Bhutani S. Worldwide burden of diabetes. Indian Journal of Endocrinology and Metabolism. 2014;18(6):868-870. d
3. American Heart Association. Cardiovascular Disease & Diabetes, 2012, http://www.heart.org/HEARTORG/Conditions/Diabetes/WhyDiabetesMatters/Cardiovascular-Disease-Diabetes_UCM_313865_Article.jsp/
4. Wilson PW, D'Agostino RB, Levy D, Belanger AM, Silbershatz H, Kannel WB. Prediction of coronary heart disease using risk factor

categories. Circulation.1998;97:1837–1847.; Wilson PW. Diabetes mellitus and coronary heart disease. Am J Kidney Dis.1998; 32:S89–S100.

5. Geiss LS, Herman WH, Smith PJ, National Diabetes Data Group. Diabetes in America. Bethesda, Md: National Institutes of Health, National Institute of Diabetes and Digestive and Kidney Diseases; 1995:233–257.

6. Smith JW, Marcus F, Serokman R. Prognosis of patients with diabetes mellitus after acute myocardial infarction. Am J Cardiol.1984;54:718–721.

7. Spector KS. Diabetic cardiomyopathy. Clin Cardiol. 1998;21:885–887.

8. Stamler J, Vaccaro O, Neaton JD, Wentworth D. Diabetes, other risk factors, and 12-year cardiovascular mortality for men screened in the Multiple Risk Factor Intervention Trial (MRFIT). Diabetes Care. 1993;16:434–444.

21. DRUGS: RECREATIONAL

Introduction

It is estimated that almost 1 in 4 people in developed countries have used recreational drugs at some time during their life. Drug abuse has now reached endemic proportions in some of these countries. Besides the social and economic impact, drug abuse has created havoc on the health care systems. There is a high rate of drug related deaths in young people.[1] Cardiovascular system damage often plays a critical role in these deaths.[2] Heroin, cocaine and amphetamines are the most common illegal drugs used in the United States.

Scientific Evidence

- Heroin (a semisynthetic analogue of morphine) is a narcotic analgesic that is commonly abused by oral ingestion, smoking or by an intravenous injection. Heroin abuse may be responsible for almost half of the drug related deaths in some countries.[3]

- Heroin increases the parasympathetic activity and reduces the sympathetic activity – this results in slow heart rate, low blood pressure and often irregular heart rhythms. Life threatening bacterial infection of the valves of the heart due to intravenous narcotic misuse is often seen. Heroin overdose may also cause the lungs to fill up with fluid (non-cardiogenic pulmonary edema) – another potentially fatal condition.[4]

- Cocaine ingestion may raise the levels of circulating catecholamines by as much as 5 times.[5] It does this by both a peripheral action (inhibiting norepinephrine reuptake in peripheral sympathetic nerve terminals) as well as a central action (stimulating central sympathetic outflow).[6] The resultant high sympathetic activity may lead to coronary artery spasms, myocardial infarction and death. Irregular heart rhythms, a dilated cardiomyopathy and non-cardiogenic pulmonary edema may also occur.[7] Sudden cardiac death has also been reported.

- Amphetamines abuse can cause similar cardiovascular complications as cocaine.[8]

Conclusion

Recreational drug abuse is a growing problem in many developed countries. The commonly used drugs, however, are extremely dangerous to the cardiovascular system and their use results in a high number of premature deaths. Certain associations maintain helpful websites. These include the American Society of Addiction Medicine [9] and the American Academy of Addiction Psychiatry.[10]

Lifestyle Implications

Stay away from recreational drug use.

References

1. Oyefeso A, Ghodse H, Clancy C, Corkery J, Goldfinch R. Drug abuse-related mortality: a study of teenage addicts over a 20-year period. Soc Psychiatry Psychiatr Epidemiol. 1999 Aug; 34(8):437-41.
2. Ghuran A, van der Wieken LR, Nolan J. Cardiovascular complications of recreational drugs: Are an important cause of morbidity and mortality. BMJ: British Medical Journal. 2001;323(7311):464-466.
3. Ghodse H, Oyefeso A, Hunt M, Pollard M, Mehta R, Corkery J. Drug related deaths as reported by the coroners in England and Wales Annual Review 1999. London: Centre for Addiction Studies, St. George's Hospital Medical School; 2000.
4. Osterwalder JJ. Patients intoxicated with heroin or heroin mixtures: how long should they be monitored? Eur J Emerg Med. 1995 Jun; 2(2):97-101.
5. Mouhaffet A, Madu EC, Satmary W, Fraker TD. Cardiovascular complication of cocaine. Chest. 1995;107:1426–1434.
6. Vongpatanasin W, Mnsour Y, Chavoshan B, Arbique D, Victor RG. Cocaine stimulates the human cardiovascular system via a central mechanism of action. Circulation. 1999 Aug 3; 100(5):497-502.
7. Ghuran A, Nolan J. Recreational drug misuse: issues for the cardiologist. Heart. 2000 Jun; 83(6):627-33.
8. Ghuran A, Nolan J. The cardiac complications of recreational drug use. Western Journal of Medicine. 2000;173(6):412-415.
9. https://www.asam.org/
10. https://www.aaap.org/

22. E-CIGARETTES

Introduction

Cigarettes are the number one cause of preventable death in the United States, killing 480,000 people every year. Smoking increases the risk of stroke, heart attack, chronic obstructive pulmonary disease, asthma, diabetes, and many cancers. The free radicals in cigarette smoke physically age the human body. On an average, smoking reduces the human life span by about 10 years. Electronic cigarettes (e-cigarettes) are less lethal than conventional cigarettes. An e-cigarette contains a cartridge of fluid, popularly known as e-liquid. E-liquid is made up of nicotine and flavorings dissolved in propylene glycol and glycerol. Nicotine is a known for its harmful effects. The e-liquid is superheated by a battery-powered vaporizer, converting it into a mist which is inhaled, or "vaped." The popularity of e-cigarettes is on the rise. The percentage of US adults who use e-cigs rose to 8.5 percent in 2013 from 3.3 percent in 2010. And in 2014, nearly 13 percent of adults said they had tried electronic cigarettes, according to the Centers for Disease Control and Prevention. More than 3 million US teens also vaped in 2015, a tenfold increase over four years. US Surgeon General, Dr. Vivek Murthy, called e-cigarettes a public health crisis. E-cigarette 'vaping' is harmful to the cardiovascular system.[1]

Scientific Evidence

- In a study of 40 healthy participants, smoking e-cigarettes decreased the bioavailability of nitric oxide and the antioxidant vitamin E – resulting in a decreased flow mediated dilation. These changes are harmful for proper endothelial function of the vessels.[2]
- In a study of 42 e-cigarette smokers, researchers found increases in low-density lipoprotein (bad) cholesterol. They also found an abnormal heart rate variability - a measure indicating sympathetic predominance. Low-density lipoprotein oxidizability, was also significantly increased in e-cigarette users, indicating increased oxidative stress.[3]
- In an analysis of the 2014 National Health Interview Survey database, researchers found that electronic cigarette use, when

adjusted for other risk factors, was associated with a 42 % increased risk of myocardial infarction.[4]

Conclusion

Electronic cigarettes are promoted as smoking cessation tools and are considered safer than regular cigarettes. Electronic cigarettes do not contain tobacco and do not involve combustion, and are therefore considered safe to smoke. However, they do contain the addictive nicotine and some of the toxic and cancer-causing chemicals found in regular cigarettes. Nicotine can elevate adrenaline levels and increase sympathetic activity. E-cigarette users have sympathetic predominance and increased oxidative stress, indicating an increased cardiovascular risk.

Lifestyle Implications

E-cigarettes may be tried for smoking cessation, under the supervision of your health care provider. Remember, they contain nicotine, an addicting compound.

References

1. Bhatnagar A. Are Electronic Cigarette Users at Increased Risk for Cardiovascular Disease? JAMA Cardiol. 2017;2(3):237–238.
2. Carnevale R, Sciarretta S, Violi F, et al. Acute Impact of Tobacco vs Electronic Cigarette Smoking on Oxidative Stress and Vascular Function. Chest. 2016 Sep;150(3):606-12.
3. Roya S. Moheimani, May Bhetraratana, Fen Yin, Kacey M. Peters, Jeffrey Gornbein, Jesus A. Araujo, Holly R. Middlekauff. Increased Cardiac Sympathetic Activity and Oxidative Stress in Habitual Electronic Cigarette Users" Implications for Cardiovascular Risk. JAMA Cardiol. Published online February 1, 2017.
4. Nardos Temesgen, Ivan Pena, Tahir Tayeb, Talal Alzahrani. A cross sectional study reveals an association between electronic cigarette use and myocardial infarction. Poster, GW Annual Research Days 2017.

23. EGGS

Introduction

Eggs from domesticated chickens have been eaten as food in South East Asia and India before 7500 BCE.[1] Eggs are a good source of antioxidants such as carotenoids, healthy essential fatty acids, choline and many vitamins and minerals. The egg yolk is high in cholesterol (approximately 200 mg per egg). Though the entire egg is edible, the egg shell is rarely consumed, despite its high calcium content. Common culinary use of egges is as boiled, omelet, scrambled, fried, and pickled. They are also used in many cooked dishes, including baked goods and desserts.

Scientific Evidence

- High cholesterol levels have been tied to cardiovascular disease.[2]
- Cholesterol lowering leads to a major reduction in cardiovascular events.[3] It has been recommended, by several professional associations in the past, that the intake of eggs should be limited, due to their high cholesterol content and their potential negative impact on cardiovascular disease.[4]
- However, recent studies have questioned the egg cholesterol – cardiovascular disease connection Most recent studies have found that the intake of one egg per day does not appear to affect the cholesterol profile deleteriously.[5]
- Eggs are nutrition dense and besides cholesterol, contain many healthy vitamins and minerals. Eggs also tend to raise the protective high-density lipoprotein cholesterol levels. Eggs are also rich in cardiovascular beneficial antioxidants.
- In a study of 37,851 men aged 40 to 75 years at study outset and 80,082 women aged 34 to 59 years at study outset, and free of cardiovascular disease, diabetes, hypercholesterolemia, or cancer, researchers found that consumption of up to 1 egg per day did not have any substantial impact on the risk of coronary heart disease or stroke. They found that eating one egg per day is safe for healthy men and women.[6]
- In another large study of 33,994 men and women free of cardiovascular disease, conducted in the USA from 1988 to 1994,

with follow-up through 31 December 2000, researchers found no increase in cardiovascular risk with eating one egg a day.[7]

- A recent meta-analysis also suggests that egg intake of up to 1 per day may reduce the incidence of stroke.[8]

Conclusion

Eating one egg per day appears to be risk free for most healthy individuals. If there is heart disease or diabetes, the data on moderate egg consumption (one per day) and an increase in heart disease is suggested but not conclusive. Suggestions that eating eggs may reduce strokes appears to have more support by evidence based data. The new 2015-2020 dietary guidelines from the U.S. Department of Health and Human Services and U.S. Department of Agriculture do not mention a daily limit on cholesterol intake.[9] The previous recommendation was to limit cholesterol intake to 300 mg/day if healthy and 200 mg /day if one had heart disease or diabetes. In patients with heart disease or diabetes, cholesterol intake may be curtailed by limiting the use of eggs or using only egg whites, which have no cholesterol. Healthier eggs are also on the horizon. These eggs will have higher omega 3 fatty acids and lower cholesterol and lower saturated fats – and may be considered as functional foods, when available.

Lifestyle Implications

It is safe to eat one egg a day without worrying about your cholesterol level – if you are otherwise healthy.

References

1. Wikepedia: https://en.wikipedia.org/wiki/Egg_as_food
2. Critchley J, Liu J, Zhao D, Wei W, Capewell S. Explaining the increase in coronary heart disease mortality in Beijing between 1984 and 1999. Circulation. 2004 Sep 7;110(10):1236-44. Epub 2004 Aug 30.
3. Cholesterol Treatment Trialists' (CTT) Collaborators. The effects of lowering LDL cholesterol with statin therapy in people at low risk of vascular disease: meta-analysis of individual data from 27 randomised trials. Lancet. 2012;380(9841):581-590.
4. Krauss RM, Eckel RH, Howard B, Appel LJ, Daniels SR, Deckelbaum RJ, et al. AHA Dietary Guidelines: revision 2000: a statement for healthcare professionals from the Nutrition Committee of the Am Heart Association. Stroke 2000; 31:2751-66.

5. Fernandez ML, Calle M. Revisiting dietary cholesterol recommendations: does the evidence support a limit of 300 mg/d? Curr Atheroscler Rep. 2010 Nov;12(6):377-83.

6. Frank B. Hu, MD; Meir J. Stampfer, MD, et al. A Prospective Study of Egg Consumption and Risk of Cardiovascular Disease in Men and Women. JAMA. 1999;281(15):1387-1394.

7. Scrafford CG, Tran NL, Barraj LM, Mink PJ. Egg consumption and CHD and stroke mortality: a prospective study of US adults. Public Health Nutr. 2011 Feb;14(2):261-70. doi: 10.1017/S1368980010001874. Epub 2010 Jul 16.

8. Alexander DD, Miller PE, Vargas AJ, Weed DL, Cohen SS. Meta-analysis of Egg Consumption and Risk of Coronary Heart Disease and Stroke. J Am Coll Nutr. 2016 Nov-Dec;35(8):704-716. Epub 2016 Oct 6.

9. Health guidelines 2015:
http://health.gov/dietaryguidelines/2015/guidelines/

24. ENERGY DRINKS

Introduction

Energy drinks contain stimulants to increase mental (memory, alertness and mood) performance.[1] Their consumption also results in an increase in physical endurance.[2] Increased focus and decreased fatigue have also been reported.[3] They usually contain caffeine, sugars, herbal extracts, taurine, and amino acids. Caffeine, a natural stimulant, is the main active ingredient and most energy drinks contain 80–150 mg of caffeine per 8 ounces.[4] Although popular, especially in college campuses, they are not without damaging health effects. These include damaging neurological,[5] gastro-intestinal,[6] renal,[7] and dental effects.[8] Their use in children is also a major concern.[9] Detrimental cardiovascular effects have been reported with their consumption.[10]

Scientific Evidence

- Energy drinks can increase the heart rate and raise the arterial blood pressure.[11]
- Habitual use may increase caloric intake and result in obesity.[12]
- Irregular heart rhythms have been reported.[13]
  Abnormal vascular endothelial function has been seen[14] and other arterial vascular damages have also been reported.[15]

Conclusion

Energy drinks can temporarily improve mental and physical alertness and endurance. Their use is common all over the world, especially in athletes, for improving performance in sports activities. It is estimated that energy drinks are consumed by 30% to 50% of all adolescents and young adults. However, excess consumption may lead to cardiovascular damage, especially in adolescents. The American Academy of Pediatrics does not recommend that energy drinks be consumed by children and adolescents.

Lifestyle Implications

Avoid or be cautious if consuming energy drinks.

References

1. Alford C, Cox H, Wescott R. The effects of red bull energy drink on human performance and mood. Amino Acids. 2001;21(2):139–150.
2. Hoffman JR, Kang J, Ratamess NA, Hoffman MW, Tranchina CP, Faigenbaum AD. Examination of a pre-exercise, high energy supplement on exercise performance. J Int Soc Sports Nutr. 2009; 6:2.
3. Walsh AL, Gonzalez AM, Ratamess NA, Kang J, Hoffman JR. Research article Improved time to exhaustion following ingestion of the energy drink. Amino Impact™ 2010.
4. Alsunni AA, Badar A. Energy drinks consumption pattern, perceived benefits and associated adverse effects amongst students of University of Dammam, Saudi Arabia. J Ayub Med Coll Abbottabad. 2011 Jul-Sep;23(3):3–9.
5. Bedi N, Dewan P, Gupta P. Energy drinks: Potions of illusion. Indian pediatrics. 2014;51(7):529–533.
6. Vivekanandarajah A, Ni S, Waked A. Acute hepatitis in a woman following excessive ingestion of an energy drink: a case report. J Med Case Rep. 2011;5(227):8.
7. Riesenhuber A, Boehm M, Posch M, Aufricht C. Diuretic potential of energy drinks. Amino Acids. 2006 Jul;31(1):81–83.
8. Hasselkvist A, Johansson A, Johansson A-K. Dental erosion and soft drink consumption in Swedish children and adolescents and the development of a simplified erosion partial recording system. Swedish dental journal. 2009;34(4):187–195.
9. Wolk B. J., Ganetsky M., Babu K. M. Toxicity of energy drinks. Current Opinion in Pediatrics. 2012;24(2):243–251.
10. Goldfarb M, Tellier C, Thanassoulis G. Review of published cases of adverse cardiovascular events after ingestion of energy drinks. The American journal of cardiology. 2014;113(1):168–172.
11. Bell DG, Bordeleau JMR, Jacobs I. Blood pressure and heart rate after caffeine and ephedrine ingestion. Can J Appl Physiol. 1999;24(5):426.
12. Moreno MA, Furtner F, Frederick PR. Sugary drinks and childhood obesity. Arch Pediatr Adolesc Med. 2009;163(4):400.
13. Di Rocco JR, During A, Morelli PJ, Heyden M, Biancaniello TA. Atrial fibrillation in healthy adolescents after highly caffeinated beverage consumption: two case reports. J Med Case Reports. 2011;5(1):18.
14. Pommerening MJ, Cardenas JC, Radwan ZA, Wade CE, Holcomb JB, Cotton BA. Hypercoagulability after energy drink consumption. Journal of Surgical Research. 2015.
15. González W, Altieri P, Alvarado E, Banchs H, Colón E, Escobales N, et al. Celiac trunk and branches dissection due to energy drink consumption and heavy resistance exercise: case report and review of literature. Boletin de la Asociacion Medica de Puerto Rico. 2014;107(1):38–40.

25. EXERCISE: AEROBIC

Introduction

Exercise is good for the human health. The famed Indian physician Susruta in 600 BC, prescribed exercise to his patients. Hippocrates (460–377 BC) praised the health benefits of physical exercise. Both Plato (427–347 BC) and Galen (129–217 AD) referred to exercise as an important complement to medicine and important for maintaining good health.[1] Leisure time physical activity is especially important for a healthy cardiovascular system, and is associated with about a 30-50% reduction in risk of coronary heart disease.

Scientific Evidence

- Several large and well conducted scientific studies have demonstrated the cardiovascular protective effects of regular physical exercise.[2] In the MRFIT Study, leisure time exercise reduced cardiovascular mortality (during a 16 year follow up) in men with a high risk of coronary heart disease.[3] The Honolulu Heart Study, documented that elderly men walking more than 1.5 miles per day reduced their risk of coronary disease. Physical activity was also associated with cardio-protection in the Nurses' Health Study and the Iowa Study.[4]

- There is a reduction in blood pressure with exercise.[5] The lipid profile is improved with a reduction in triglyceride levels, increase in high-density lipoprotein cholesterol levels and a decrease in the low-density lipoprotein to high-density lipoprotein ratio.[6] Obesity is reduced. Exercise improves sugar metabolism and insulin sensitivity,[7] and reduces systemic inflammation.[8] There is an improvement in autonomic tone,[9] decrease in blood coagulation,[10] enhanced endothelial function,[11] and improved coronary blood flow and heart function.

- Many psychological risk factors (stress, anxiety and depression) for cardiovascular diseases are also improved by routine physical activity.[12]

- Even low levels of exercise, especially in the old and frail, have cardiovascular benefits.[13]

Conclusion

The American Heart Association recommends at least 150 minutes per week of moderate exercise (thirty minutes a day, five times a week) or 75 minutes per week of vigorous exercise (or a combination of moderate and vigorous activity) for cardiovascular health benefits. In elderly and otherwise frail populations, even lower levels of exercise impart cardiovascular health benefits.

Lifestyle Implications

Partake in regular physical exercise during your leisure time. Every physical activity counts towards maintaining a well working cardiovascular system and prevents future cardiovascular diseases.

References

1. Agarwal SK. Cardiovascular benefits of exercise. International Journal of General Medicine. 2012;5:541-545.
2. S. Goya Wannamethee, A. Gerald Shaper. Physical Activity and Cardiovascular Disease. Seminars in Vascular Medicine 2002; 02(3): 257-266.
3. Leon AS, Myers MJ, Connett J. Leisure time physical activity and the 16-year risks of mortality from coronary heart disease and all-causes in the MRFIT. Int J Sports Med. 1997 Jul;18: S208–S215.
4. Hakim AA, Curb JD, Petrovitch H, et al. Effects of walking on coronary heart disease in elderly men: the Honolulu Heart Program. Circulation. 1999. 100 (1):9-13.
5. Blair SN, Goodyear NN, Gibbons LW, et al. Physical fitness and incidence of hypertension in healthy normotensive men and women. JAMA 1984;252:487-90.
6. Berg A, Halle M, Franz I, et al. Physical activity and lipoprotein metabolism: epidemiological evidence and clinical trials. Eur J Med Res 1997;2:259-64
7. Wallberg-Henriksson H, Rincon J, Zierath JR. Exercise in the management of non-insulin-dependent diabetes mellitus. Sports Med 1998;25:25-35.
8. Adamopoulos S, Parissis J, Kroupis C, et al. Physical training reduces peripheral markers of inflammation in patients with chronic heart failure. Eur Heart J 2001;22:791-7.
9. Tiukinhoy S, Beohar N, Hsie M. Improvement in heart rate recovery after cardiac rehabilitation. J Cardiopulm Rehabil 2003;23:84-7.

10. Rauramaa R, Salonen JT, Seppanen K, et al. Inhibition of platelet aggregability by moderate-intensity physical exercise: a randomized clinical trial in overweight men. Circulation 1986;74:939-44.

11. Gokce N, Vita JA, Bader DS, et al. Effect of exercise on upper and lower extremity endothelial function in patients with coronary artery disease. Am J Cardiol 2002;90:124-7.

12. Dunn AL, Trivedi MH, O'Neal HA. Physical activity dose–response effects on outcomes of depression and anxiety. *Med Sci Sports Exerc* 2001;33:S587-97.

13. Leon AS, Connett J, Jacobs DR Jr., et al. Leisure-time physical activity levels and risk of coronary heart disease and death. The Multiple Risk Factor Intervention Trial. JAMA 1987;258:2388-95.

26. EXERCISE: RESISTANCE

Introduction

The cardiovascular benefits of resistance exercise (such as lifting weights) are not well recognized by the general public. A loss of muscle mass and a decrease in the quality of skeletal muscle, has been recognized as increasing the cardiovascular risk, especially in the aging population.[1] This increase in risk can be prevented or reversed by regular resistance training.[2] Resistance exercise results in an improvement of several cardiovascular risk factors,[3] and a reduction in the risk of coronary heart disease by 23%.[4]

Scientific Evidence

- In multivariate analyses, researchers found that that weight training for 30 minutes or more per week was associated with a 23% risk reduction in coronary heart disease.[4]
- In a large cross-sectional analysis which included 7,321 women with no history of heart disease, hypertension or diabetes, researchers found that resistance exercise independently improved cardiovascular risk profiles in these women.[5]
- Several cardiovascular risk factors are improved by resistance training,[6] including a reduction in blood pressure,[7] improvement in glucose metabolism,[8] and a bettering of the lipid profile.[9]
- Resistance training helps increase resting metabolic rate and improve fat free mass.[10] Metabolic syndrome is reduced.[11]
- Resistance exercise helps improve mental health, including depression and anxiety.[12]

Conclusion

The American Heart Association recommends strength training along with endurance, flexibility and balance exercises, for cardiovascular protection. Strength or resistance training should be done at least twice per week. Strength training can be done with free weights (such as barbells and dumbbells), ankle cuffs and vests, resistance (elastic) bands or by using your own body weight against gravity.

Lifestyle Implications

Adding weight or resistance training to the aerobic work routine not only strengthens the musculoskeletal system but also enhances cardiovascular benefits. Ideally, resistance exercises should be done two times a week.

References

1. Strasser B, Siebert U, Schobersberger W. Resistance training in the treatment of the metabolic syndrome: a systematic review and meta-analysis of the effect of resistance training on metabolic clustering in patients with abnormal glucose metabolism. Sports Med. 2010;40(5):397–415.

2. Williams MA, Haskell WL, Ades PA, et al. Resistance exercise in individuals with and without cardiovascular disease: 2007 update: a scientific statement from the American Heart Association Council on Clinical Cardiology and Council on Nutrition, Physical Activity, and Metabolism. Circulation. 2007;116(5):572–584.

3. Artero EG, Lee DC, Lavie CJ, et al. Effects of muscular strength on cardiovascular risk factors and prognosis. J Cardiopulm Rehabil Prev. 2012;32(6):351–358.

4. Tanasescu M, Leitzmann MF, Rimm EB, Willett WC, Stampfer MJ, Hu FB. Exercise Type and Intensity in Relation to Coronary Heart Disease in Men. *JAMA*. 2002;288(16):1994-2000.

5. Drenowatz C, Sui X, Fritz S, et al. The association between resistance exercise and cardiovascular disease risk in women. Journal of science and medicine in sport / Sports Medicine Australia. 2015;18(6):632-636.

6. Cornelissen VA, Fagard RH, Coeckelberghs E, et al. Impact of resistance training on blood pressure and other cardiovascular risk factors: a meta-analysis of randomized, controlled trials. Hypertension. 2011;58(5):950–958.

7. Hurley BF, Roth SM. Strength training in the elderly. Sports Med. 2000;30:249-268.

8. Poehlman ET, Dvorak RV, DeNino WF, Brochu M, Ades PA. Effects of resistance training and endurance training on insulin sensitivity in nonobese, young women. J Clin Endocrinol Metab.2000;85:2463-2468.

9. Prabhakaran B, Dowling EA, Branch JD, Swain DP, Leutholtz BC. Effect of 14 weeks of resistance training on lipid profile and body fat percentage in premenopausal women. Br J Sports Med.1999;33:190-195.

10. Poehlman ET, Melby C. Resistance training and energy balance. Int J Sport Nutr.1998;8:143-159.

11. Jurca R, Lamonte MJ, Barlow CE, et al. Association of muscular strength with incidence of metabolic syndrome in men. Med Sci Sports Exerc. 2005;37(11):1849–1855.

12. http://www.heart.org/HEARTORG/HealthyLiving/PhysicalActivity/Fit
nessBasics/Strength-and-Resistance-Training-
Exercise_UCM_462357_Article.jsp#.WP-16tLys1I)

27. EXERCISE: STRETCHING

Introduction

Cardiorespiratory fitness is a combination of muscular strength, aerobic endurance, and flexibility. Stretching improves flexibility. Stretching exercises are widely used for injury protection, but they are also good for optimal cardiovascular health.[1] Good flexibility is an indicator of preserved vascular elasticity,[2] and correlates well with cardiorespiratory fitness.[3] Increased arterial stiffness (lack of vascular elasticity) is an independent risk factor for mortality and cardiovascular events.[4]

Scientific Evidence

- In a study of 526 adults, researchers found that a less flexible body indicated arterial stiffening, especially in middle-aged and older adults.[2]
- Arterial stiffness is associated with increased cardiovascular events, especially in the older population.[5]
- Stretching improves the cardiovascular beneficial parasympathetic tone.[6]
- Stretching exercises for ten minutes, done before bedtime, result in a decrease in depression.[7] Depression is linked with an increase in cardiovascular diseases.

Conclusion

Besides aerobic and resistance training, stretching exercises aimed at improving flexibility reduce arterial stiffness and result in decreased cardiovascular events. The American Heart Association recommends several stretching exercises to increase flexibility and maintain cardiovascular health. These include torso stretch and torso twist for the midsection, neck stretch for the cervical area, seated march for hip flexibility, quadriceps stretch for the front thigh muscles and hamstring stretch for the back-thigh muscles.[8]

Lifestyle Implications

Incorporate stretching exercises to improve your flexibility, in addition to endurance and resistance exercises – for optimal cardiovascular fitness.

References

1. American College of Sports Medicine Position Stand (ACSM). Quantity and quality of exercise for developing and maintain cardiorespiratory, musculoskeletal, and neuromotor fitness in apparently healthy adults: Guidance for prescribing exercise. Med Sci Sport Exerc. 2011;43:1334-1359.
2. Kenta Yamamoto, Hiroshi Kawano, Yuko Gando, et al. Poor trunk flexibility is associated with arterial stiffening. American Journal of Physiology - Heart and Circulatory Physiology Published 1 October 2009 Vol. 297 no. 4, H1314-H1318.
3. Vaitkevicius PV, Fleg JL, Engel JH, et al. Effects of age and aerobic capacity on arterial stiffness in healthy adults. Circulation 88: 1456–1462, 1993.
4. Laurent S, Boutouyrie P, Asmar R, Gautier I, Laloux B, Guize L, Ducimetiere P, Benetos A. Aortic stiffness is an independent predictor of all-cause and cardiovascular mortality in hypertensive patients. Hypertension 37: 1236–1241, 2001.
5. Sutton-Tyrrell K, Najjar SS, Boudreau RM, et al. Elevated aortic pulse wave velocity, a marker of arterial stiffness, predicts cardiovascular events in well-functioning older adults. Circulation 111: 3384–3390,2005.
6. Farinatti PT, Brandão C, Soares PP, Duarte AF. Acute effects of stretching exercise on the heart rate variability in subjects with low flexibility levels. J Strength Cond Res. 2011 Jun;25(6):1579-85.
7. Kai Y, Nagamatsu T, Kitabatake Y, Sensui H. Effects of stretching on menopausal and depressive symptoms in middle-aged women: a randomized controlled trial. Menopause. 2016 Aug;23(8):827-32.
8. http://www.heart.org/HEARTORG/Conditions/More/CardiacRehab/Stretching-and-Flexibility-Exercises_UCM_307383_Article.jsp#.WP_RAdLys1I.

28. FATS

Introduction

Unsaturated fats are usually liquid at room temperature and include monounsaturated fats and polyunsaturated fats. They contain a double bond within the fatty acid chain – monounsaturated have one double bond while polyunsaturated have more than one double bond. A high number of double bonds makes the fat more vulnerable to lipid peroxidation (leading to rancidity). Saturated fats have no double bonds and are saturated with hydrogen atoms. They are therefore less vulnerable to rancidity and are favored in processed foods. Saturated fats are more solid at room temperature than unsaturated fats. Omega-3 fats are polyunsaturated fats come from food sources and are heart healthy. Trans fats are made by hydrogenation of vegetable oils – making them more stable. They are commonly used in the food industry for frying and in baked goods and processed snack foods. Margarine is made from trans fats. Trans fats are heart unhealthy.

Scientific Evidence

- Polyunsaturated fats reduce coronary heart disease.[1] They decrease low-density lipoprotein cholesterol levels and raise high-density lipoprotein cholesterol levels.[2] In a recent study, a diet predominantly rich in monounsaturated fats, lowered blood pressure, improved lipid levels, and reduced overall cardiovascular risk.[3]

- Omega-3 fatty acids are plentiful in fish – and an adequate supply is obtained by eating fish 2-3 times a week. Flax seeds, walnuts, and canola or soybean oil, are also good sources of omega-3. Research has shown that omega-3 fatty acids lower the risk of arrhythmias, decrease triglyceride levels, slow growth rate of atherosclerotic plaque, and slightly lower blood pressure.[4] They also reduce inflammation - fish eaters have a lower incidence of coronary artery disease.[5,6]

- Saturated fats are heart unhealthy. Major dietary sources of saturated fats are pizza, cheese, whole milk, butter, cookies, dairy desserts and meat products such as sausage, bacon, beef, and hamburgers. However recent reports have questioned the validity of the cardiovascular dangers associated with saturated fats. A meta-analysis of twenty-one studies, with 347,747 subjects showed that intake of saturated fat did not increase the risk of coronary heart disease, stroke or cardiovascular diseases. This study had a 5-23 year follow up, during which period 11,006 participants developed coronary heart disese or stroke.[7]

- Trans fats raise low-density lipoprotein cholesterol and lower the high-density lipoprotein cholesterl levles. They also create inflammation and increase insulin resistance – conditions that are detrimental to the cardiovascular system. It is estimated that a 2% daily increase in the intake of calories from tans fats increases the risk of coronary heart disease by 23%. Trans fats are being gradually eliminated from the foods, as per a ban announced by the FDA in June 2015.

Conclusion

Several cardiovascular guidelines encourage high consumption of foods rich in polyunsaturated fatty acids (avocado, nuts, canola, sunflower, flaxseed and olive oils, and fish) and low consumption of foods high in saturated fats. Food made with trans fats should be avoided. The 2015-2020 Dietary Guidelines recommend keeping saturated fat consumption to less than 10% of total calories consumed per day and encourage replacing saturated fat with unsaturated fat.[8] Replacing saturated fat with carbohydrates does not provide cardiovascular benefits.

Lifestyle Implications

Cut down on saturated fat and replace it with unsaturated fat in your diet. Your heart and blood vessels will thank you.

References

1. Mozaffarian, D., R. Micha, and S. Wallace, Effects on coronary heart disease of increasing polyunsaturated fat in place of saturated fat: a systematic review and meta-analysis of randomized controlled trials. PLoS Med, 2010. 7(3): p. e1000252.
2. Mensink, R.P., et al., Effects of dietary fatty acids and carbohydrates on the ratio of serum total to HDL cholesterol and on serum lipids and apolipoproteins: a meta-analysis of 60 controlled trials. Am J Clin Nutr, 2003. 77(5): p. 1146-55.

3. Appel, L.J., et al., Effects of protein, monounsaturated fat, and carbohydrate intake on blood pressure and serum lipids: results of the OmniHeart randomized trial. JAMA, 2005. 294(19): p. 2455-64.

4. http://www.heart.org/HEARTORG/HealthyLiving/HealthyEating/HealthyDietGoals/Fish-and-Omega-3-Fatty-Acids_UCM_303248_Article.jsp#.WY96YlGGMcw

5. Ascherio A, Rimm EB, Stampfer MJ, Giovannucci EL, Willett WC. Dietary intake of marine n-3 fatty acids, fish intake, and the risk of coronary disease among men. N Engl J Med. 1995;332:977–982.

6. Hu FB, Bronner L, Willett WC, et al. Fish and omega-3 fatty acid intake and risk of coronary heart disease in women. JAMA. 2002;287:1815–1821.

7. Siri-Tarino PW, Sun Q, Hu FB, Krauss RM. Meta-analysis of prospective cohort studies evaluating the association of saturated fat with cardiovascular disease. The American Journal of Clinical Nutrition. 2010;91(3):535-546.

8. https://www.choosemyplate.gov/2015-2020-dietary-guidelines-answers-your-questions

29. FIBER

Introduction

Dietary fiber is derived from plants, and is indigestible. It can be soluble or insoluble. The soluble fiber absorbs water and gives a feeling of fullness after eating, Insoluble fiber does not dissolve in water. It helps soften the stool, and its bulking action eases defecation. Several studies have shown that soluble fiber reduces several risk factors for cardiovascular diseases.

Scientific Evidence

- A cross-sectional analysis of 23,168 men and non-pregnant women aged 20+ years from the 1999–2010 National Health and Nutrition Examination Survey revealed that higher dietary fiber intake was associated with a lower prevalence of cardiometabolic risks.[1]
- The beneficial effect of increased fiber intake on blood pressure has been noted in several studies.[2,3] Although the blood pressure reductions are small, they do translate into appreciable long-term cardiovascular risk reduction.
- In a meta-analysis of 67 controlled trials, soluble fiber decreased both total as well as the 'bad' low-density lipoprotein cholesterol.[4]
- Researchers found an inverse association between dietery fiber intake and serum C-reactive protein concentration (CRP - a biomarker of inflammation) when they studied data from the National Health and Nutrition Examination Survey 1999-2000. This study included 3,920 participants who were 20 or more years old.[5] Similar findings have been reported by other investigators[6]
- Studies have also noted a decrease in other risk factors, including the metabolic syndrome, obesity,[7] and impaired insulin sensitivity[8,9] in people with high fiber intake.

Conclusion

According to the Institute of Medicine,[10] adequate intake for total fiber is 38 grams and 25 grams per day for men (age 14-50 years) and women (age 19-50 years), respectively. After age 50, men need 30 grams and women need 21 grams per day of total fiber. Soluble fiber is found in fruits (such as apples, oranges and grapefruit), vegetables, legumes (such as dry beans, lentils and peas), barley, oats and oat bran. Insoluble fiber is found in fruits with edible peel, seeds, vegetables, whole grain products (such as whole-wheat bread, pasta and crackers), wheat, stone ground corn meal, cereals, bran, rolled oats, buckwheat and brown rice.

Lifestyle Implications

Increasing your intake of whole grains, legumes, fruits and vegetables should give you adequate fiber and help decrease several risk factors for cardiovascular diseases.

References

1. Grooms KN, Ommerborn MJ, Pham DQ, Djousse L, Clark CR. Dietary Fiber Intake and Cardiometabolic Risks among US Adults, NHANES 1999–2010. The American journal of medicine. 2013;126(12): 10.1016/j.amjmed.2013.07.023.
2. He J, Whelton PK, Klag MJ. Dietary fiber supplementation and BP reduction: a meta-analysis of controlled trials. Presented at the 16th Scientific Meeting of the International Society of Hypertension, Glasgow, UK, 1996.
3. Valerie Burke, Jonathan M. Hodgson, Lawrie J. Beilin, Nella Giangiulioi, Penny Rogers and Ian B. Puddey. Dietary Protein and Soluble Fiber Reduce Ambulatory Blood Pressure in Treated Hypertensives. Hypertension. 2001;38:821-826.
4. Brown L, Rosner B, Willett WW, Sacks FM. Cholesterol-lowering effects of dietary fiber: a meta-analysis. Am J Clin Nutr. 1999;69(1):30–42.
5. Ajani, U.A., Ford, E.S., and Mokdad, A.H. Dietary fiber and C-reactive protein: findings from national health and nutrition examination survey data. J Nutr. 2004; 134: 1181–1185.
6. King, D.E., Egan, B.M., and Geesey, M.E. Relation of dietary fat and fiber to elevation of C-reactive protein. Am J Cardiol. 2003; 92: 1335–1339.
7. Slavin, J.L. Position of the American Dietetic Association: health implications of dietary fiber. J Am Diet Assoc. 2008; 108: 1716–1731.
8. Schneeman, B.O. Dietary fiber and gastrointestinal function. Nutr Rev. 1987; 45: 129–132.
9. Liese, A.D., Schulz, M., Fang, F. et al. Dietary glycemic index and glycemic load, carbohydrate and fiber intake, and measures of insulin sensitivity, secretion, and adiposity in the Insulin Resistance Atherosclerosis Study. Diabetes Care. 2005; 28: 2832–2838.
10. Institute of Medicine. 2005. Dietary Reference Intakes for Energy, Carbohydrate, Fiber, Fat, Fatty Acids, Cholesterol, Protein, and Amino Acids. National Academy Press. (Food and Nutrition Board, Institute of Medicine, National Academies).

30. FISH

Introduction

According to Wikipedia, there are over 33,000 species of fish. Fishes are cold blooded and usually covered with scales. They breathe by taking oxygen from the water, using gills. Several fishes are popular as human food and these include carp, cod, herring, perch, sardines, sturgeon, tilapia, trout, and tuna. Fish consumption per capita has been increasing worldwide, from an average of 9.9 kg in the 1960s to almost 16.4 kg in 2005. Fish is a good source of protein and contains many vitamins and minerals. It is low in saturated fat. The Inuit population of Greenland consumes primarily whales, seals, sea birds, and fish and have a low incidence of ischemic heart disease. This has been attributed to the marine-derived omega-3 polyunsaturated fatty acids, namely, eicosapentaenoic acid and docosahexaenoic acid.[1] A large study suggested that consumption of one to two 3-ounce servings of fatty fish a week could reduce the risk of dying from heart disease by 36% and total mortality by 17%.[2]

Scientific Evidence

- Omega-3 fatty acids improve several cardiometabolic risk factors including abnormal lipids, high blood pressure, increased vascular reactivity and poor cardiac function. They also have cardioprotective anti-thrombotic, anti-inflammatory and anti-oxidative properties.[3]
- In a study of older adults (3,326 US men and women age ≥65 years), higher circulating long-chain n-3 polyunsaturated fatty acids and docosahexaenoic acid - both high in fish, were associated with lower risk of incident atrial fibrillation. Atrial fibrillation causes irregular and rapid heart-beats which increase the risk of stroke, heart failure and other heart-related complications.[4]
- Eating fish (one to two 3-ounce servings of fatty fish a week - salmon, herring, mackerel, anchovies, or sardines) reduces heart disease mortality by 36% and total mortality by 17%.[2]

Conclusion

High levels of fish intake may be one factor explaining the lowest coronary heart disease mortality and longest life expectancy among developed countries, in the Japanese.[5]

Lifestyle Implications

Incorporate fish as part of a healthy diet. Eat approximately one to two 3-ounce servings of fatty fish a week—salmon, herring, mackerel, anchovies, or sardines. You will live longer.

References

1. Bang HO, Dyerberg J, Nielsen AB. Plasma lipid and lipoprotein pattern in Greenlandic West-coast Eskimos. Lancet. 1971 Jun 5; 1(7710):1143-5.
2. Mozaffarian D, et al "Fish Intake, Contaminants, and Human Health: Evaluating the Risks and the Benefits" JAMA. 2006; 296:1885-1899.
3. Mori TA. Omega-3 fatty acids and cardiovascular disease: epidemiology and effects on cardiometabolic risk factors. Food Funct. 2014 Sep;5(9):2004-19.
4. Jason H.Y. Wu, Rozenn N. Lemaitre, Association of Plasma Phospholipid Long-Chain Omega-3 Fatty Acids with Incident Atrial Fibrillation in Older Adults: The Cardiovascular Health Study. Circulation, August 8, 2017, Volume 136, Issue 6.
5. Yamori Y, Sagara M, Arai Y, Kobayashi H. Soy and fish as features of the Japanese diet and cardiovascular disease risks. PLoS One. 2017 Apr 21;12(4): e0176039.

31. FRUITS

Introduction

Regular fruit intake is associated with a lower incidence of several diseases and promotes a longer life span.[1] Fruit consumption is also associated with decreased risks of cardiovascular disease,[2] and cardiovascular mortality.[3]

Scientific Evidence

- In a large study from China, involving 512,891 persons, a 40% lower risk of cardiovascular death and a 34% lower risk of major coronary events was noted among participants who consumed fresh fruit daily, when compared to those who never or rarely consumed fresh fruit.[4]

- A Cochrane review of 10 trials with a total of 1,730 participants, and one ongoing trial, concluded that increased intake of fruits (and vegetables) has favorable effects on cardiovascular risk factors.[5] Several other large studies and reviews have reached similar conclusions.[6]

- Fruits are low in sodium, fat and calories. They are rich in several minerals, vitamins, fiber and bioactive compounds with potential cardioprotective effects.[7] These include anti-oxidant,[8] hypo-lipidemic,[9] and anti-platelet actions.[10]

- They also help reduce several conventional cardiovascular risk factors such as hypertension,[11] diabetes,[12] and obesity.[13]

- Cardiovascular mortality is reduced with fruit consumption. The risk of all-cause mortality, including cardiovascular mortality, may be decreased by about 6% with fruit consumption.[14]

Conclusion

The beneficial relationship between fruit intake and a reduced cardiovascular disease and cardiovascular mortality is persuasive. Raw fruit is higher in dietary fiber than fruit juices, which may also be altered during processing.[15] Most studies, however, show benefits of fruit intake, irrespective of it being consumed raw or as 100% juice, on the cardiovascular system.

Lifestyle Implications

Incorporate fruits in your daily diet. Theoretically, raw and richly colored fruits may be slightly more cardioprotective.

References

1. Genkinger JM, Platz EA, Hoffman SC, Comstock GW, Helzlsouer KJ. Fruit, vegetable, and antioxidant intake and all-cause, cancer, and cardiovascular disease mortality in a community-dwelling population in Washington County, Maryland. Am J Epidemiol. 2004;160.12:1223–33.
2. Bazzano LA, He J, Ogden LG, Loria CM, Vupputuri S, Myers L, et al. Fruit and vegetable intake and risk of cardiovascular disease in US adults: the first National Health and Nutrition Examination Survey Epidemiologic Follow-up Study. Am J Clin Nutr. 2002;76.1:93–9.
3. Okuda N., Miura K., Okayama A., et al. Fruit and vegetable intake and mortality from cardiovascular disease in Japan: A 24-year follow-up of the NIPPON DATA80 study. Eur. J. Clin. Nutr. 2015;69:482–488.
4. Du H, Li L, Bennett D, et al. Fresh Fruit Consumption and Major Cardiovascular Disease in China. The New England journal of medicine. 2016;374(14):1332-1343.
5. Hartley L, Igbinedion E, Holmes J, et al. Increased consumption of fruit and vegetables for the primary prevention of cardiovascular diseases. Cochrane Database Syst Rev. 2013;6:CD009874.
6. Oyebode O, Gordon-Dseagu V, Walker A, Mindell JS. Fruit and vegetable consumption and all-cause, cancer and CVD mortality: analysis of Health Survey for England data. J Epidemiol Community Health. 2014;68:856–62.
7. Liu RH. Health benefits of fruit and vegetables are from additive and synergistic combinations of phytochemicals. Am J Clin Nutr. 2003;78(Suppl):517S–20S.
8. Fu L., Xu B.T., Xu X.R., et al. Antioxidant capacities and total phenolic contents of 62 fruits. Food Chem. 2011;129:345–350.
9. Aiso I, Inoue H, Seiyama Y, Kuwano T. Compared with the intake of commercial vegetable juice, the intake of fresh fruit and komatsuna (Brassica rapa L. var. perviridis) juice mixture reduces serum cholesterol in middle-aged men: a randomized controlled pilot study. Lipids in Health and Disease. 2014;13:102.
10. Assefa AD, Ko EY, Moon SH, Keum Y-S. Antioxidant and antiplatelet activities of flavonoid-rich fractions of three citrus fruits from Korea. 3 Biotech. 2016;6(1):109.

11. Du H., Li L., Bennett D., et al. Fresh fruit consumption, blood pressure and cardiovascular disease risk: A prospective cohort study of 0.5 million adults in the China kadoorie biobank. Eur. Heart J. 2014;351:725.

12. Cooper AJ, Sharp SJ, Lentjes MA, Luben RN, Khaw KT, Wareham NJ, et al. A prospective study of the association between quantity and variety of fruit and vegetable intake and incident type 2 diabetes. Diabetes Care 2012;35:1293-300.

13. Bazzano LA, Serdula MK, Liu S. Dietary intake of fruits and vegetables and risk of cardiovascular disease. Curr Atheroscler Rep. 2003;5:492–9.

14. Wang X, Ouyang Y, Liu J, et al. Fruit and vegetable consumption and mortality from all causes, cardiovascular disease, and cancer: systematic review and dose-response meta-analysis of prospective cohort studies. The BMJ. 2014;349: g4490.

15. Barrett DM, Lloyd B. Advanced preservation methods and nutrient retention in fruits and vegetables. J Sci Food Agric 2012;92:7–22.

32. FRUIT JUICE

Introduction

It is well known that consumption of fruits is associated with a decreased risk of cardiovascular disease.[1] The US Department of Health and Human Services recommends that adults who engage in <30 minutes of moderate physical activity daily should consume 1.5–2.0 cup equivalents of fruit daily.[2] Fruit juices are a convenient way of meeting the fruit recommendations. Epidemiologic and other clinical evidence suggests a beneficial association between intake of certain fruit juices, their polyphenolic compounds; and a better cardiovascular health.[3] 100% fruit juice is considered equivalent to one cup of fruit. Currently, in the US, only 32% of adults and 13% of adolescents meet this goal of fruit intake.[4] Despite this poor compliance, recent recommendations advocate increasing fruit consumption even more, given their persuasive health benefits.

Scientific Evidence

- Fruit intake helps keep blood pressure lower.[5] Several fruit juices, especially pomegranate juice, guava fruit juice and cherry juice may help reduce both systolic and diastolic blood pressure.
- Some fruit juices like apple juice, berry juice, tomato juice may help improve the lipid profile, such as lower serum low-density lipoprotein cholesterol, lower total cholesterol, and lower triglycerides.[3] Fruits also help decrease low-density lipoprotein cholesterol oxidation,[6] improve vascular function,[7] and increase arterial blood flow.[6]
- Platelets play an important role in the development of atherosclerotic cardiovascular complications. Both orange juice and grape juice inhibit platelet aggregation.[8]
- Persistent inflammation is negatively related to cardiovascular diseases. Many fruit juices, especially plum, peach, cranberry and red orange, attenuate cardiovascular inflammation.[9]

Conclusion

100% fruit juice has many cardiovascular benefits because of their high phytochemical content. Grapejuice, promegate juice and cranberry juice may be more cardioprotective as they contain more beneficial compounds than other fruit juices. Adding berries, especially, blackberry, black raspberry, blueberry, cranberry, red raspberry, and strawberries to these juices greatly increases their cardiovascular beneficial properties. Berries are low in calories and are high in moisture, fiber, vitamins and micronutrients besides the beneficial bioactive phytochemicals. Drinking juice with pulp increases the amount of fiber taken in, further enhancing cardiac health. Fruit juices taken in excess over the recommended limits may cause more harm than good, due to their high glycemic sugar and caloric content. Sweetened fruit juices should be avoided. According to the American Academy of Pediatrics, intake of fruit juice should be limited to 4 to 6 oz/day in children 1 to 6 years old. For children 7 to 18 years old, juice intake should be limited to 8 to 12 oz or 2 servings per day.[10]

Lifestyle Implications

Drinking unsweetened fruit juice (preferably a cocktail made from several fruits, including berries) with pulp, is beneficial for cardiovascular health.

References

1. Okuda N., Miura K., Okayama A., et al. Fruit and vegetable intake and mortality from cardiovascular disease in Japan: A 24-year follow-up of the NIPPON DATA80 study. Eur. J. Clin. Nutr. 2015;69:482–488.
2. USDA and US Department of Health and Human Services. Dietary guidelines for Americans, 2010. 7th ed. Washington (DC): US Government Printing Office; 2010.
3. Zheng J, Zhou Y, Li S, et al. Effects and Mechanisms of Fruit and Vegetable Juices on Cardiovascular Diseases. Speranza L, Franceschelli S, eds. International Journal of Molecular Sciences. 2017;18(3):555.
4. Centers for Disease Control and Prevention. The Youth Risk Behavior Surveillance System (YRBSS) Atlanta: Centers for Disease Control and Prevention; 2007.
5. Asgary S., Sahebkar A., Afshani M.R., et al. Clinical evaluation of blood pressure lowering, endothelial function improving, hypolipidemic and anti-Inflammatory effects of pomegranate juice in hypertensive subjects. Phytother. Res. 2014;28:193–199.
6. Stein JH, Keevil JG, Wiebe DA, Aeschlimann S, Folts JD. Purple grape juice improves endothelial function and reduces the sustainability of LDL

cholesterol to oxidation in patients with coronary artery disease. Circulation 1999;100:1050–5.

7. Buscemi S, Rosafio G, Arcoleo G, Mattina A, Canino B, Montana M, Verga S, Rini G. Effects of red orange juice intake on endothelial function and inflammatory markers in adult subjects with increased cardiovascular risk. Am J Clin Nutr 2012;95:1089–95.

8. Napoleone E., Cutrone A., Zurlo F., et al. Both red and blond orange juice intake decreases the procoagulant activity of whole blood in healthy volunteers. Thromb. Res. 2013;132:288–292.

9. Buscemi S, Rosafio G, Arcoleo G, Mattina A, Canino B, Montana M, Verga S, Rini G. Effects of red orange juice intake on endothelial function and inflammatory markers in adult subjects with increased cardiovascular risk. Am J Clin Nutr 2012;95:1089.

10. http://pediatrics.aappublications.org/content/107/5/1210.

33. GARDENING

Introduction

Gardening is an extremely popular leisure activity all over the world. It is estimated that in the UK, 27 million people, approximately 40% of the total population, actively participate in gardening.[1] Likewise, it is estimated that in the US, 117 million people, or one in three, participate in gardening. In Japan, 32 million people, or one in four, participate in daily gardening as a hobby. Gardening is a good non-exercise physical activity, with several health benefits.[2] It is also cardio-protective.

Scientific Evidence

- Regular exercise protects against cardiovascular disease.[3] Gardening involves moderate-intensity physical activity with upper and lower body movement, and may help adults achieve recommended physical activity levels.[4] Gardening may also encourage people to undertake other physical exercise.[5]
- Gardening improves depression and anxiety symptoms, stress, mood disturbance, and body weight - factors that modulate cardiovascular diseases.[6]
- Gardening also results in an improved cardiovascular profile. In a study published in the British Journal of Sports Medicine, 4,232 individuals in Stockholm County were followed for an average of 12.5 years, for cardiovascular disease events and mortality. In this group, people with high levels of non-exercise physical activity (NEPA), when compared with to people with low NEPA, had a better waist circumference, better high-density lipoprotein cholesterol and triglyceride levels in both sexes and lower insulin, glucose and fibrinogen levels in men. High NEPA level, compared with low, was associated with a lower risk of a first cardiovascular event and lower all-cause mortality.[7]
- Daily gardening "for pleasure" also implies motivation and happiness – positive cardioprotective emotions.[8] Gardening also reduces social isolation - anothr risk factor for cardiovascular disease.[9]

- Gardening will indirectly encourage a healthier diet, with home grown fruits and vegetables. A diet rich in fruits and vegetables is cardio-protective.[10]
- Gardening also reduces overall mortality. In a Taiwanese study of 5,058 adults over 50 years in age with mobility limitations, daily home gardening as a leisure-time activity decreased mortality by about 18%.[11]

Conclusion

Gardening is a feasible leisure time activity at any age, and is especially cardioprotective in older adults. Cardiovascular benefits accrue from gardening related physical activity, generation of mentally uplifting emotions, improvement in social interactions and the increased intake of fresh fruits and vegetables.

Lifestyle Implications

Gardening should be done by all individuals, and especially middle-aged and older adults, as a leisure activity, Gardening can be done in the backyard, in a community lot or even in the apartment, with significant cardiovascular benefits.

References

1. Bisgrove R., Hadley P. UK Climate Impacts Programme; Oxford, UK: 2002. Gardening in the Global Greenhouse: The Impacts of Climate Change on Gardens in the UK.
2. Wang D., MacMillan T. The benefits of gardening for older adults: a systematic review of the literature. Act. Adapt. Aging. 2013;37:153–181.
3. Park SA, Lee KS, Son KC, Shoemaker CA. Metabolic cost of horticulture activities in older adults. J Japan Soc Hort Sci. 2012;81(3):295–299.
4. Zick C.D., Smith K.R., Kowaleski-Jones L., Uno C., Merrill B.J. Harvesting more than vegetables: the potential weight control benefits of community gardening. Am. J. Public Health. 2013;103:1110–1115.
5. Soga M, Gaston KJ, Yamaura Y. Gardening is beneficial for health: A meta-analysis. Preventive Medicine Reports. 2017;5:92-99.
6. E. Ekblom-Bak, B. Ekblom, M. Vikstrom, U. de Faire, M.-L. Hellenius. The importance of non-exercise physical activity for cardiovascular health and longevity. British Journal of Sports Medicine, 2013.

7. Clayton S. Domesticated nature: motivations for gardening and perceptions of environmental impact. J Environ Psychol. 2007;27:215–224.

8. Hartig T, Mitchell R, de Vries S, Frumkin H. Nature and health. Annu Rev Public Health. 2014;35:207–228.

9. Clatworthy J, Hinds J, Camic PM. Gardening as a mental health intervention: a review. Ment Health Rev (Brighton) 2013;18(4):214–225.

10. Wang X, Ouyang Y, Liu J, et al. Fruit and vegetable consumption and mortality from all causes, cardiovascular disease, and cancer: systematic review and dose-response meta-analysis of prospective cohort studies. The BMJ. 2014;349:g4490.

11. Lêng CH, Wang J-D. Daily home gardening improved survival for older people with mobility limitations: an 11-year follow-up study in Taiwan. Clinical Interventions in Aging. 2016;11:947-959.

34. GARLIC

Introduction

Garlic (*Allium sativum*) originated in Central Asia. It has a pungent flavor, and is used all over the world as a seasoning or condiment. Garlic cloves are consumed raw, pickled or cooked. About 65% of garlic is water, while the rest is composed of fructose-containing carbohydrates, sulfur compounds, protein, fiber, and free amino acids.[1] Garlic is also rich in saponins, phosphorus, potassium, sulfur, zinc, moderate levels of selenium and vitamins A and C. It has small amounts of calcium, magnesium, sodium, iron, manganese, and B-complex vitamins. It also contains a significant amount of several antioxidant phenolic compounds.[2] Garlic has been used for medicinal purposes for centuries, especially in China and India.[3] Egyptian tomb carvings from 3,700 BC, also indicate its medicinal use. Diseases treated included tumors and headaches. Garlic may be beneficial in preventing cardiovascular diseases.[4]

Scientific Evidence

- Hypercholestrolemia is a major cause of coronary heart disease and lowering blood cholesterol levels, with statin drugs, has been associated with a decrease in cardiovascular disease. In a meta-analysis of several studies, researchers concluded that garlic, in an amount approximating one half to one clove per day, decreased total serum cholesterol levels by about 9% in the patients (with cholesterol levels above 200 mg/dl) studied.[5] Other studies have confirmed the cholesterol reducing effects, although modest, of garlic.[6] Alder and associates included 10 studies in a review and found that in 6 studies garlic was effective in reducing not only the total serum cholesterol levels by about 9.9%, but also low-density lipoprotein cholesterol by 11.4%, and triglycerides by 9.9%.[7]

- Oxidation of low-density lipoprotein cholesterol is also a major contributor to the development of atherosclerosis.[8] Atherosclerosis is a major cause of cardiovascular diseases. Garlic may reduce atherosclerosis by inhibiting the oxidation of low-density lipoprotein cholesterol and thus help prevent cardiovascular disease.[9]

- Garlic extracts help lower blood pressure.[10]

- Garlic extract also has anti-oxidant activity and decreases platelet aggregation.[11]

Conclusions

Garlic and aged garlic extract have several properties and actions that help reduce cardiovascular diseases.

Lifestyle Implications

Make garlic a regular condiment in your cooking.

References

1. Lawson LD. The composition and chemistry of garlic cloves and processed garlic. In Koch HP, Lawson LD, editors. Garlic the science and therapeutic application of *Allium sativum L* and related species. (Baltimore: Williams & Wilkins; 1996. p. 37–107.
2. Vinson JA, Su X, Zubik L, Bose P. Phenol antioxidant quantity and quality in foods: fruits. J Agric Food Chem. 2001;49:5315–21.
3. Block, E. (1985) The chemistry of garlic and onion. Sci. Am. 252:114-119.
4. Banerjee SK, Maulik SK. Effect of garlic on cardiovascular disorders: a review. Nutr J. 2002;1:4–14.
5. Warshafsky S, Kamer RS, Sivak SL. Effect of Garlic on Total Serum Cholesterol: A Meta-Analysis. Ann Intern Med. 1993;119:599-605.
6. Stevinson C, Pittler MH, Ernst E. Garlic for treating hypercholesterolemia. A meta-analysis of randomised clinical trials. Ann Intern Med. 2000;19:420–9.
7. Alder R, Lookinland S, Berry JA, Williams M. A systematic review of the effectiveness of garlic as an antihyperlipidemic agent. J Am Acad Nurse Pract.2003;15:120–9.
8. Cox, D. A. & Cohen, M. L. (1996) Effects of oxidized low density lipoproteins on vascular contraction and relaxation: clinical and pharmacological implications in atherosclerosis. Pharmacol. Rev. 48:3-9.
9. Lau, Benjamin HS, Moses A. Adetumbi, and Albert Sanchez. "Allium sativum (garlic) and atherosclerosis: a review." Nutrition research 3.1 (1983): 119-128.
10. Sendl A, Elbl G, Steinke B, Redl K, Breu W, Wagner H. Comparative pharmacological investigations of *Allium ursinum* and *Allium sativum*. Planta Med. 1992;58:1–7.
11. Durak I, Kavutcu M, Aytac B, Avci A, Devrim E, Ozbek H, Ozturk HS. Effects of garlic extract consumption on blood lipid and oxidant/antioxidant parameters in humans with high blood cholesterol. J Nutr Biochem. 2004;15:373–7.

35. GINGER

Introduction

Ginger is the rhizome of the perennial plant, Zingiber officinale. Ginger was originally called 'smagaveram' – a Sanskrit name meaning 'horn root', based on its appearance. It has been called ziggiberis in Greek and Zinziberi in Latin. It is one of the most commonly consumed dietary condiments in the world.[1] Its characteristic aroma is mainly due to ketones, especially gingerols. Powdered dry ginger root is often used to flavor gingerbread, cookies, crackers, cakes, ginger ale, and ginger beer. It has also been used by the Indians and Chinese during the past 5000 years, for its several medicinal properties, including its cardioprotective actions.

Scientific Evidence

- Oxidation of the circulating low-density lipoprotein cholesterol plays a causal role in atherosclerosis, which is the underlying pathology leading to heart attacks and ischemic strokes.[2]
- Antioxidant nutrients inhibit these damaging oxidative processes and are believed to slow the progression of atherosclerosis.[3]
- However, this anti-oxidant benefit does not appear to work with anti-oxidant vitamins. In a review of 22 trials, researchers concluded that antioxidant vitamins do not appear to provide protection against cardiovascular disease.[4]
- Futher, several large-scale studies have found that supplemental intake of some vitamins with significant anti-oxidant properties such as beta-carotene, vitamin A, and vitamin E may actually increase mortality.[5]
- However, naturally occurring antioxidants in fruits and vegetables, appear to be beneficial for prevention of atherosclerosis and decrease cardiovascular disease and cardiovascular mortality.[6]
- This anti-oxidant activity is primarily dependent on their high content of phenolic compounds.[7] Flavonoids constitute a major part of these antioxidant compounds.
- Ginger is rich in flavonoids. The main antioxidants in ginger are gingerols and some related phenolic ketone derivatives.[8] Ginger is therefore considered a good food for the prevention of atherosclerosis and its progression.[9]

- Ginger is also beneficial against cardiovascular diseases in many other ways. Its extracts in rat studies have demonstrated an improvement in lipid levels.[10] A good lipid profile is cardiovascular friendly.

- Ginger may also have some hypotensive, anti-inflammatory and anti-platelet effects.[11] These effects are again cardiovascular friendly.

- Ginger may also have anti-diabetic effects.[12] Diabetes is a major risk factor for cardiovascular disease.

Conclusion

Ginger due to its high phenolic content, may have cardiovascular protective effects. It is a heart healthy condiment to have in the kitchen. Ginger use is generally safe, although it may cause heartburn or interfere with anti-coagulants. Reports that it may interfere with diabetes or blood pressure medications are rarely seen in real life.

Lifestyle Implications

Like garlic, ginger should be in every kitchen, and used regularly in cooking.

References

1. Surh Y. J. Molecular mechanisms of chemopreventive effects of selected dietary and medicinal phenolic substances. Mutat Res. 1999;428(1-2):305–27.
2. Ross R. Atherosclerosis—an inflammatory disease. N Engl J Med 1999;340:115–26.
3. Parthasarathy S. Mechanisms by which dietary antioxidants may prevent cardiovascular diseases. J Med Food 1998;1:45–51.
4. Katsiki N, Manes C. Is there a role for supplemented antioxidants in the prevention of atherosclerosis? Clin Nutr. 2009;28:3–9.
5. Bjelakovic G, Nikolova D, Gluud C. Antioxidant supplements and mortality. Curr Opin Clin Nutr Metab Care. 2014;17:40–44.
6. Kaliora AC, Dedoussis GV, Schmidt H. Dietary antioxidants in preventing atherogenesis. Atherosclerosis. 2006 Jul;187(1):1-17.
7. Marja P. Ka¨hko¨nen, Anu I. Hopia, et al. Antioxidant Activity of Plant Extracts Containing Phenolic Compounds. J. Agric. Food Chem. 1999, 47, 3954–3962.
8. Zachariah TJ. Ginger. In: Parthasarathy VA, Champakam B, Zachariah TG, editors. Chemistry of Spices. CABI. 2008. pp. 70–100.

9. Akinyemi, Ayodele Jacob et al. Effect of Two Ginger Varieties on Arginase Activity in Hypercholesterolemic Rats. Journal of Acupuncture and Meridian Studies, 2016, Volume 9 , Issue 2 , 80 – 87.

10. Al-Noory AS, Amreen A-N, Hymoor S. Antihyperlipidemic effects of ginger extracts in alloxan-induced diabetes and propylthiouracil-induced hypothyroidism in (rats). Pharmacognosy Research. 2013;5(3):157-161.

11. Nicoll R, Henein M. Y. Ginger (Zingiber officinale Roscoe): A hot remedy for cardiovascular disease? Int J Cardiol. 2009;131(3):408–9.

12. Islam M. S, Choi H. Comparative effects of dietary ginger (Zingiber officinale) and garlic (Allium sativum) investigated in a type 2 diabetes model of rats. J Med Food. 2008;11(1):152–9.

36. GRAPE JUICE

Introduction

Grapes, *Vitis vinifera*, have been used for their taste and their nutritional value by humans since the Neolithic period. They are now grown and consumed all over the world. Grapes, like other fruits, are heart healthy, but may have stronger protective effects. Wine is made from grapes and is considered one of the main cardiovascular protective agents in the Mediterranean diet.[1] However, many people in the world do not drink wine. Somewhat similar cardioprotective effects may be present in non-wine grape products.[2] The medicinal value of grapes and grape juice has also been recognized for over 6000 years.[3] Grapes and grape elixirs have been used therapeutically for several conditions, such as nausea, constipation, cholera, smallpox, liver and kidney diseases, and various cancers. Even sap from the grape-wines had medicinal properties and has been used as an ointment to treat skin and eye conditions.

Scientific Evidence

- Grapes, like many other fruits and vegetables, are rich in polyphenols. Anthocyanins are polyphenolic pigments, and mainly exist in red/purple grape skins and are a major anti-oxidant component of red grape juice. They help reduce atherosclerosis by several mechanisms.

- Grape polyphenol intake, in the form of grape juice, can significantly reduce the systolic blood pressure in humans.[4]

- Unlike citrus juices, grape juice also inhibits platelet aggregation.[5] Purple grape juice is rich in flavonols, anthocyanidins and proanthocyanidins,[6] with the flavonols exerting stronger anti-platelet actions than the favanones found in citrus juices.[7]

- In a study involving twenty-six patients receiving hemodialysis and 15 healthy subjects, all individuals were given 100 mL red grape juice to drink daily for 14 days and several cardiovascular biomarkers were tested regularly. Similar blood testing was done in 12 other randomly recruited hemodialysis patients not receiving the juice. The study found that dietary supplementation with concentrated red grape juice improves the lipoprotein profile, reduces plasma concentrations of inflammatory biomarkers and

97

oxidized low-density lipoprotein cholesterol. These changes are cardioprotective.[8]

- Seeds of grapes have the highest antioxidant capacity, followed by the skin. The flesh has the lowest antioxidant capacity. Researchers found that 77.3% of the phytonutrients in grapes are found in the seed, 21.6% in the skin, and only 1.1% in the pulp.[9] Grape juice made from seeded red grapes may therefore have the most cardioprotective activity.

Conclusion

Grape juice, has significant cardioprotective activity, much more than orange juice. The benefit is primarily from its phenolic compounds, which appear to be greatest in the seeds. Grape seeds contain proanthocyanidin phenols, that exert an anti-oxidant activity that is 20 times greater than vitamin E and 50 times greater than vitamin C.[10] The skin of red grapes is rich in phenolic compounds quercetin and resveratrol.

Lifestyle Implications

Unsweetened red or purple grape juice is cardioprotective.

References

1. St Leger AS, Cochrane AL, Moore F. Factors associated with cardiac mortality in developed countries with particular reference to the consumption of wine. Lancet. 1979;1:1017–20.
2. Di Castelnuovo A, Rotondo S, Iacoviello L, Donati MB, de Gaetano G. Meta-analysis of wine and beer consumption in relation to vascular risk. Circulation. 2002;105:2836–44.
3. Ziskind B, Halioua B. Occupational medicine in ancient Egypt. Med Hypotheses. 2007;69:942–5.
4. Li S-H, Zhao P, Tian H-B, Chen L-H, Cui L-Q (2015) Effect of Grape Polyphenols on Blood Pressure: A Meta-Analysis of Randomized Controlled Trials. PLoS ONE 10(9): e0137665. https://doi.org/10.1371/journal.pone.0137665
5. Jon G. Keevil, Hashim E. Osman, Jess D. Reed, and John D. Folts. Grape Juice, But Not Orange Juice or Grapefruit Juice, Inhibits Human Platelet Aggregation. J. Nutr. January 1, 2000 vol. 130 no. 1 53-56.
6. Silva, J.M.R., Riguld, J., Cheynier, V., Cheminat, A. & Moutounet, M. (1991) Procyanidin dimers and trimers from grape seeds. Phytochemistry 30:1259-1264.

7.   Landolfi, R., Mower, R. L. & Steiner, M. (1984) Modification of platelet function and arachidonic acid metabolism by bioflavonoids. Structure-activity relations. Biochem. Pharmacol. 33:1525-1530.

8.   Patricia Castilla, Rocío Echarri, Alberto Dávalos, et al. Concentrated red grape juice exerts antioxidant, hypolipidemic, and antiinflammatory effects in both hemodialysis patients and healthy subjects. Am J Clin Nutr. 2006 Jul;84(1):252-62.

9.   Ivanova V, Stefova M, Chinnici F. Determination of the polyphenol contents in Macedonian grapes and wines by standardized spectrophotometric methods. J Serb Chem Soc. 2010;75:45–59.

10. Shi J, Yu J, Pohorly JE, Kakuda Y (2003). "Polyphenolics in grape seeds-biochemistry and functionality". J Med Food. 6 (4): 291–9.

37. HAPPINESS

Introduction

Happiness is being satisfied with your life and feeling good every day. Being happy is an important objective of life. Happiness appears to depend both on inherited factors as well as on external or environmental factors. Research suggests that true happiness is determined by a combination of both factors. Genes, especially *5-HTTLPR* and *MAOA*. have an influence of about 33%, on our happiness.[1] Exogenous factors include a multitude of behavioral, socio-cultural, economical, and geographical life events. Physical health, attractiveness and quality of life also play a major role. Although money helps to live a better life, it does not necessary correlate with happiness. Happiness is good for your heart health!

Scientific Evidence

- Happy people tend to be healthier and live longer. Decreased cardiovascular mortality is one reason for this longevity.

- People with happiness also behave healthier – they maintain healthy lifestyles when compared to those that are unhappy. Healthier life styles correlate with less cardiovascular disease. Happier people shy away from risky behaviors. They smoke less and drink less – factors that negatively influence cardiovascular diseases.

- Happy people are less likely to become obese.[2] Obesity is linked with cardiovascular disease. Happy societies tend to have less high blood pressure among its inhabitants.[3] High blood pressure is a major contributor to the pathogenesis of cardiovascular disease.

- Mental stress is known to induce ischemia in patients with coronary artery disease,[4] and contributes to an increased mortality in these patients. Perceived mental stress is also associated with increased mortality from stroke in women. Happy people are less burdened by mental stress.

- Depression and a loss of sense of purpose in life is associated with increased cardiovascular disease. Negative emotions such as hostility and anxiety are also associated with an increase in cardiovascular events. Happy people have less negativity.

- In a study evaluating the sense of purpose in life, done in 1988, a prospective cohort of 2,959 Japanese subjects, ranging in age from 40 to 74 years, were followed till the end of 2003, with deaths and their causes recorded. The level of their sense of purpose in life was evaluated by a self-administered questionnaire. [5] Researchers found that having a strong sense of purpose in life, an essential part of satisfaction and happiness, was associated with reduced cardiovascular events, especially in men.

- Researchers examined the association between positive affect and cardiovascular events in 1,739 adults (862 men and 877 women) in the 1995 Nova Scotia Health Survey. Data showed a healthy positive affect was protective against 10-year incident coronary heart disease.[6]

- Positivity, especially happiness, is associated with many neuro-hormonal changes that are cardioprotective. These include lower blood pressure, better sleep, lower norepinephrine levels and better heart rate variability in people. The protective para-sympathetic tone is also increased.

- In a major review from the Harvard School of Public Health, published in 2012, researchers concluded that positive psychological well-being was good for cardiovascular health.[7]

Conclusion

Positive emotions include joy, happiness, excitement, enthusiasm, and contentment. Several recent scientific studies have confirmed that negative emotions such as hostility, anxiety and depression worsen the risk of getting or aggravating cardiovascular disease, and are associated with increased mortality. Happiness on the other hand, tends to provide a protective effect. Since a major aspect of the emotion of happiness is based on non-genetic factors, moving your mental balance towards being happy, having a purpose in life, excitement and contentment, will induce mental and physical changes that will be cardio-protective.

Lifestyle Implications

Death is inevitable. So why worry? Be Happy!

References

1. De Neve J-E, Christakis NA, Fowler JH, Frey BS. Genes, Economics, and Happiness. Journal of neuroscience, psychology, and economics. 2012;5(4):10.1037/a0030292.

2. El Shebini LS, Kazem YMI, Moaty MIA, El-Arabi NHA. (2011). Obesity in Relation to Cognitive Functions and Subjective Wellbeing among a Group of Adult Egyptian Females. Aus J Basic Appl Sci, 5(6): 69–76.

3. Blanchflower DG, Oswald AJ (2007). Hypertension and Happiness across Nations. United Kingdom, University of Warwick, Department of Economics.

4. Krantz DS, Sheps DS, Carney RM, Natelson BH. Effects of mental stress in patients with coronary artery disease: evidence and clinical implications. JAMA 2000;283:1800-2.

5. Koizumi M, Ito H, Kaneko Y, Motohashi Y. Effect of Having a Sense of Purpose in Life on the Risk of Death from Cardiovascular Diseases. Journal of Epidemiology. 2008;18(5):191-196.

6. Davidson KW, Mostofsky E, Whang W. Don't worry, be happy: positive affect and reduced 10-year incident coronary heart disease: The Canadian Nova Scotia Health Survey. European Heart Journal. 2010;31(9):1065-1070.

7. Julia K. Boehm and Laura D. Kubzansky. The Heart's Content: The Association Between Positive Psychological Well-Being and Cardiovascular Health. Psychological Bulletin. 2012, Vol. 138, No. 4, 655–691.

38. HEIGHT

Introduction

Short people have a higher risk for the development of coronary artery disease.[1] Height is a non-modifiable risk factor for cardiovascular disease. This genetic relationship is however not well known. Short people should therefore take other risk factors for coronary artery disease even more seriously, and be more diligent in following cardiovascular healthy lifestyles.

Scientific Evidence

- Shorter adult height is associated with an increased risk of coronary artery disease.[2]
- An earlier study documented that every inch of added height results in an approximate 2% to 3% decline in the risk of myocardial infarction. Researchers found this unique association in a study of 22,071 male physicians.[3]
- Shorter people have an increased incidence of several cardiovascular risk factors, including hypertension, high levels of low-density lipoprotein cholesterol and diabetes.[4]
- Shorter people have coronary arteries with smaller diameter and this may contribute to the higher cardiovascular risk.[5]
- An inverse relationship has also been noted with stroke.[6,7]
- Several other cardiovascular diseases also have a curious relationship to height. Taller individuals tend to have more atrial fibrillation, mitral valve prolapse and Marfan's syndrome. Shorter people have more congestive heart failure and aortic valve calcification.[8]

Conclusion

An inverse relationship exists between height and several cardiovascular risk factors and coronary artery disease. The connection appears to be genetically determined.

Lifestyle Implications

Although tall people are not immune from coronary artery disease, being shorter should induce a more diligent compliance with healthy heart lifestyles.

References

1. Christopher P. Nelson, Ph.D., Stephen E. Hamby, Ph.D., Danish Saleheen, et al. Genetically Determined Height and Coronary Artery Disease. N Engl J Med 2015; 372:1608-1618.
2. Paajanen TA, Oksala NKJ, Kuukasjarvi P, Karhunen PJ. Short stature is associated with coronary heart disease: a systematic review of the literature and a meta-analysis. Eur Heart J 2010;31:1802-1809.
3. P R Hebert, J W Rich-Edwards, J E Manson, et al. Height and incidence of cardiovascular disease in male physicians. Circulation. 1993;88:1437-1443.
4. Gunnell D, Whitley E, Upton MN, McConnachie A, Smith GD, Watt GC. Associations of height, leg length, and lung function with cardiovascular risk factors in the Midspan Family Study. J Epidemiol Community Health 2003;57:141-146.
5. O'Connor NJ, Morton JR, Birkmeyer JD, Olmstead EM, O'Connor GT. Effect of coronary artery diameter in patients undergoing coronary bypass surgery. Circulation 1996;93:652-655.
6. Hozawa A, Murakami Y, Okamura T, Kadowaki T, Nakamura K, Hayakawa T, Kita Y, Nakamura Y, Okayama A, Ueshima H. Relation of adult height with stroke mortality in Japan. NIPPON DATA80. Stroke. 2007;38:22–26.
7. Honjo K, Iso H, Inoue M, Tsugane S. Adult height and risk of cardiovascular disease among middle aged men and women. Eur J Epidemiol. 2011;26:13–21.
8. Rosenbush SW, Parker JM. Height and heart disease. Rev Cardiovasc Med. 2014;15(2):102-8.

39. HIGH BLOOD PRESSURE

Introduction

Normal blood pressure is defined as levels of less than 120 mm Hg systolic or 80 mm Hg diastolic. Blood pressure levels between 120 and 139 mm Hg systolic or 80 to 89 mm Hg diastolic refer to pre-hypertension. High blood pressure is defined as a systolic blood pressure of at least 140 mm Hg or a diastolic blood pressure of at least 90 mm Hg. High blood pressure is often without symptoms. It is estimated that more than 65% of adults in the United States have blood pressure levels higher than normal. Its prevalence rises dramatically with increasing age; the lifetime probability of developing hypertension is perhaps as high as 90%.[1] Black race/ethnicity persons have higher blood pressure levels than persons of white race/ethnicity, resulting in a higher cardiovascular mortality in the former.[2] Although the data reveals that hypertension is strongly associated with an increased risk of cardiovascular disease and cardiovascular mortality,[3] less than 50% of hypertensives are controlled to levels below 140/90 mm Hg, despite the use of medications.[4] Controlling high blood pressure in hypertensives reduces their risk of developing heart disease and stroke, however, this risk still remains higher than in those who have a normal blood pressure level naturally.

Scientific Evidence

- People with pre-hypertension have a 1.5 to 2.5 times greater risk of having a heart attack, a stroke, or heart failure in 10 years than those with normal blood pressure levels.[5]
- For every increase of 20 mm Hg in systolic blood pressure above 115/75 mm Hg, the risk of death from coronary heart disease and stroke doubles.[6]
- Hypertension is a major cause of heart failure. The Systolic Hypertension in Elderly Program trial (4,736 people >60 years of age) demonstrated that reducing blood pressure from 170/77 to 143/78 mm Hg reduced heart failure events by 48%.[7]
- Hypertension is also a major cause of cardiac arrhythmias. Besides symptoms, irregular heart rhythm is dangerous and may result in strokes or sudden death.[8]

Conclusion

Hypertension is a somewhat preventable disease. Preventing or controlling high blood pressure will protects against cardiovascular events and premature mortality. The guidelines of the National Heart, Lung, and Blood Institute recommend the following 5 approaches to prevent hypertension: (1) reduction of sodium intake, (2) weight reduction in persons who are overweight, (3) regular physical activity, (4) moderation of alcohol intake, and (5) an eating plan that is rich in fruits, vegetables, and low-fat dairy products and reduced in saturated fat, total fat, and cholesterol.[9]

Lifestyle Implications

Prevent getting, delay the onset or reduce the severity of high blood pressure by following the recommendations of the NHLBI and the American Heart Association. If you already suffer from hypertension, follow your health providers recommendations, for an adequate control.

References

1. Vasan RS, Beiser A, Seshadri S, et al. Residual lifetime risk for developing hypertension in middle-aged women and men: the Framingham Heart Study. JAMA. 2002;287(8):1003-1010.
2. Roger VL, Go AS, Lloyd-Jones DM, et al; American Heart Association Statistics Committee and Stroke Statistics Subcommittee. Executive summary: heart disease and stroke statistics—2012 update: a report from the American Heart Association [published correction appears in Circulation. 2012;125(22):e1001]. Circulation. 2012;125(1):188-197.
3. Chobanian AV, Bakris GL, Black HR, et al. The Seventh Report of the Joint National Committee on Prevention, Detection, Evaluation, and Treatment of High Blood Pressure: the JNC 7 report. JAMA. 2003;289:2560–2572.
4. Egan BM, Zhao Y, Axon RN. US trends in prevalence, awareness, treatment, and control of hypertension, 1988-2008. JAMA. 2010;303(20):2043-2050.
5. Vasan RS, Larson MG, Leip EP, et al. Impact of high-normal blood pressure on the risk of cardiovascular disease. N Engl J Med. 2001;345(18):1291-1297.
6. Lewington S, Clarke R, Qizilbash N, Peto R, Collins R; Prospective Studies Collaboration. Age-specific relevance of usual blood pressure to vascular mortality: a meta-analysis of individual data for one million adults in 61 prospective studies. Lancet. 2002;360(9349):1903-1913.

7.   Kostis JB, Davis BR, Cutler J, Grimm RH Jr, Berge KG, et al. (1997) Prevention of heart failure by antihypertensive drug treatment in older persons with isolated systolic hypertension. SHEP Cooperative Research Group. JAMA 278:212–216.

8.   Aidietis A, Laucevicius A, Marinskis G. Hypertension and cardiac arrhythmias. Curr Pharm Des. 2007;13(25):2545-55.

9.   Whelton PK, He J, Appel LJ, et al; National High Blood Pressure Education Program Coordinating Committee. Primary prevention of hypertension: clinical and public health advisory from the National High Blood Pressure Education Program. JAMA. 2002;288(15):1882-1888.

40. HOBBIES

Introduction

Hobbies are leisure time activities that one enjoys doing alone and also help improve one's social interactions. Hobby is a pastime that brings happiness and joy. Hobbies can include gardening, stamp collecting, photography, knitting, doing crossword puzzles etc. They act as mental tonics, and often keep one physically active. They also help one relax. Hobbies can thus help reduce cardiovascular disease by inducing relaxation, generating happiness, improving social interaction and increasing leisure time exercise.

Scientific Evidence

There is scant but still significant scientific evidence on the relationship between hobbies and cardiovascular disease.

- In a study of 121 men and women, those with hobbies showed better coronary vasculature reactivity and had lower incidence of major adverse cardiovascular events during several months of observation (average follow-up period was 916 +/- 515 days).[1]
- Psychological stress is an independent risk factor for cardiovascular disease. Persistent stress is related to coronary artery disease, fatal myocardial infarction, non-fatal myocardial infarction and cardiovascular death.[2] Hobbies are relaxing and therefore anti-stress.
- Hobbies correlate with satisfaction and happiness.[3] Happiness is a positive emotion and positive psychological well-being correlates well with a better cardiovascular health.[4]
- Social isolation is harmful to the cardiovascular system. For example, individuals with smaller social networks and fewer meaningful social connections show increased depressive symptomatology,[5] and cardiovascular risk factors, such as coronary artery calcification, increased blood glucose levels, hypertension, and diabetes.[6,7] They also have an increased cardiovascular mortality.[8] Leisure time hobbies help improve social interaction.[9]
- Many hobbies improve activity, especially in older people. Physical activity plays an important role in maintaining good cardiovascular health and is associated with reduced disease and mortality.[10]

Conclusion

Hobbies are good for cardiovascular health. They reduce emotional negativity, increase social interaction and improve physical activity.

Lifestyle Implications

Hobbies are cardiovascular protective.

References

1. Saihara K, Hamasaki S, Ishida S, Kataoka T, et al. Enjoying hobbies is related to desirable cardiovascular effects. Heart Vessels. 2010 Mar;25(2):113-20.
2. Svensson T, Kitlinski M, Engström G, et al. A genetic risk score for CAD, psychological stress, and their interaction as predictors of CAD, fatal MI, non-fatal MI and cardiovascular death. PLoS One. 2017 Apr 20;12(4): e0176029.
3. Lu L, Argyle M. Leisure satisfaction and happiness as a function of leisure activity. Gaoxiong Yi Xue Ke Xue Za Zhi. 1994 Feb;10(2):89-96.
4. Boehm JK, Kubzansky LD. The heart's content: the association between positive psychological well-being and cardiovascular health. Psychol Bull. 2012 Jul;138(4):655-91.
5. Rutledge T, Linke SE, Olson MB, Francis J, Johnson BD, Bittner V, et al. Social networks and incident stroke among women with suspected myocardial ischemia. Psychosom Med. 2008;70:282–7.
6. Rutledge T, Reis SE, Olson M, Owens J, Kelsey SF, Pepine CJ, et al. Social networks are associated with lower mortality rates among women with suspected coronary disease: The National Heart, Lung, and Blood Institute-sponsored Women's Ischemia Syndrome Evaluation study. Psychosom Med. 2004;66:882–8.
7. Kop WJ, Berman DS, Gransar H, Wong ND, Miranda-Peats R, White MD, et al. Social network and coronary artery calcification in asymptomatic individuals. Psychosom Med. 2005;67:343–52.
8. Ramsay S, Ebrahim S, Whincup P, Papacosta O, Morris R, Lennon L, et al. Social engagement and the risk of cardiovascular disease mortality: results of a prospective population-based study of older men. Ann Epidemiol. 2008;18:476–83.
9. Po-Ju Chang, Linda Wray, and Yeqiang Lin. Social Relationships, Leisure Activity, and Health in Older Adults. Health Psychology. 2014, Vol. 33, No. 6, 516 –523.
10. Alves AJ, Viana JL, Cavalcante SL, et al. Physical activity in primary and secondary prevention of cardiovascular disease: Overview updated. World Journal of Cardiology. 2016;8(10):575-583.

41. INCARCERATION

Introduction

More than 10.35 million people are in prison around the world, according to a report published by the Institute for Criminal Policy Research. USA accounts for more than 2.2 million prisoners, while there are about 1.65 million in China, 640,000 in the Russian Federation, 607,000 in Brazil, 418,000 in India, 311,000 in Thailand, 255,000 in Mexico and 225,000 in Iran. Incarceration can have significant negative physical and psychological effects on human health. The prison population is not well studied, and although mental illnesses occupy a major portion of their ill health, available data strongly indicates that a deleterious cardiovascular health is also promoted by incarceration process itself.[1]

Scientific Evidence

- Many inmates disproportionately suffer from co-morbidities such as smoking, obesity, diabetes and hypertension on entry. Many prisoners come from a low socio-economic status. Many suffer from alcohol and drug dependency. Many women and young offenders also have a higher prevalence of hypercholesterolemia.
- Further, prisons may worsen cardiovascular risk factors, including obesity due to poor diet choices available and/or chosen by the inmates,[2] lack of exercise, stress and anxiety,[3] and isolation.[4]
- Access to proper medical services may be limited while incarcerated, often due to a multitude of factors.
- Ex-prisoners also suffer from poor health, including cardiovascular disease.[5] Released inmates have high rates of poverty, unemployment, homelessness and often lack proper health insurance and medical care. This contributes to high rates of hospitalization seen in the recently released prisoners,[6] and the higher rates of death in the months following their release.[7]
- Family members of the incarcerated, especially female partners, also suffer from a worsening of their cardiovascular system, including developing obesity, and heart attack or a stroke.[8]

Conclusion

Incarceration has profound deleterious effects on the health of the incarcerated as well as their spouses. Incarcerated people generally have a poor cardiovascular health prior to incarceration, which often worsens during the incarceration. Post discharge is also a dangerous period and is associated with high rates of hospitalization and death.

Lifestyle Implications

Obviously, following the law and thereby avoiding incarceration is by far the number one practical information gleaned from the data. Proper self-care, physically and mentally, both during and after incarceration, is vital for protecting the cardiovascular system.

References

1. Binswanger IA, Stern MF, Deyo RA, Heagerty PJ, Cheadle A, Elmore JG, et al. Release from prison--a high risk of death for former inmates. N Engl J Med. 2007;356(2):157–165.
2. Eves A, Gesch B. Food provision and the nutritional implications of food choices made by young adult males, in a young offenders' institution. J Hum Nutr Diet. 2003 Jun;16(3):167-79.
3. Biggam FH, Power KG. Social support and psychological distress in a group of incarcerated young offenders. Int J Offender Ther Comp Criminol. 1997;41(3):213–230.
4. Brown S, Day A. The role of loneliness in prison suicide prevention and management. J Offender Rehabil. 2008;47(4):433–449.
5. Kinner SA, Wang EA. The case for improving the health of ex-prisoners. Am J Public Health. 2014;104(8):1352---1355.
6. Emily A. Wang, Yongfei Wang, and Harlan M. Krumholz. A High Risk of Hospitalization Following Release From Correctional Facilities in Medicare Beneficiaries: A Retrospective Matched Cohort Study, 2002 to 2010. JAMA Intern Med. 2013 September 23; 173(17): 1621–1628.
7. Zlodre J, Fazel S. All-Cause and External Mortality in Released Prisoners: Systematic Review and Meta-Analysis. American Journal of Public Health. 2012;102(12): e67-e75.
8. Lee H, Wildeman C, Wang EA, Matusko N, Jackson JS. A Heavy Burden: The Cardiovascular Health Consequences of Having a Family Member Incarcerated. American journal of public health. 2014;104(3):421-427.

42. IRON

Introduction

Iron is the second most abundant metal in the Earth's crust. It is present as a trace element in the human body, is a key component of several enzymes and is essential for many cellular processes. Iron overload has been known as a risk factor in progression of atherosclerosis.[1] It is postulated that high stored iron levels, measured by serum ferritin concentrations, may contribute to the oxidative stress and thus elevate the risk for development of atherosclerosis. Some researchers however continue to question the deleterious role of excess iron in cardiovascular disease. On the other hand, iron deficiency has also been associated with cardiovascular disease and mortality.[2]

Scientific Evidence

- Researchers in a study of 99 men in Eastern Finland, found that men with high body iron stores had a twofold to threefold increase in the risk of a first heart attack. These findings confirmed similar previous epidemiological observations. People who frequently and voluntarily donate blood have reduced body iron stores, improved vascular function, and reduced oxidative stress when compared with low-frequency donors.[3]

- In a study of 100 cancer-free patients with peripheral arterial disease (PAD) participating in the Veterans Affairs Cooperative Study #410, researchers found statistically significant associations between levels of ferritin, inflammatory biomarkers, and mortality in patients with PAD.[4] PAD is a strong marker of systemic atherosclerosis and is related to myocardial infarction, ischemic stroke, and cardiovascular death.

- In a study done in Pakistan, involving 203 consecutive acute myocardial infarction patients (146 males and 57 females; age range 18–45 years) admitted to the National Institute for Cardiovascular Diseases, Karachi, and 205 healthy controls whose gender and age (within 3 years) matched the study patients, a positive association between total body iron status and risk of a premature acute heart attack was noted.[5]

- In a study of 212 participants with coronary artery disease and 220 participants free of coronary artery disease, high iron stores, as assessed by serum ferritin levels, were associated with an increased risk of coronary artery disease. [6]
- In a large meta-analysis of 21 published studies involving 292,454 participants with an average follow-up of 10.2 years, researchers found that heme (meat based) iron absorption was primarily responsible for the iron related increase in coronary heart disease.[7]
- Iron deficiency, on the other hand, has also been associated with cardiovascular disease.[8]

Conclusion

Iron is important for normal health. Iron overload can increase atherosclerosis and lead to premature and potentially fatal coronary artery disease. Reports have also associated low serum iron stores with an increased incidence of coronary artery disease. The recommended dietary iron intake is 8 mg per day in men over the age of 19 years. Women, due to iron losses from menstruation, need 18 mg per day between the ages of 19 and 50. Women 51 years of age or older, need 8 mg/day. During pregnancy, the requirement goes up to 27 mg per day.[9]

Lifestyle Implications

Do not take iron supplements, unless advised by your health care provider. Iron accumulation in the body is associated with accelerated atherosclerosis. Similarly, if you are iron deficient, replacement under the supervision of your health care provider is important.

References

1. de Valk B, Marx JJ. Iron, atherosclerosis, and ischemic heart disease. Arch Intern Med. 1999;159(14):1542–8.
2. Hsu H.-S., Li C.-I., Liu C.-S., Lin C.-C., Haung K.-C., Li T.-C., Haung H.-Y., Lin W.-Y. Iron deficiency is associated with increased risk for cardiovascular disease and all-cause mortality in the elderly living in long-term care facilities. Nutrition. 2013;29:737–743.
3. Zheng H., Cable R., Spencer B., Votto N., Katz S.D. Iron stores and vascular function in voluntary blood donors. Arterioscler. Thromb. Vasc. Biol. 2005;25:1577–1583.
4. DePalma, Ralph G, et al. Ferritin levels, inflammatory biomarkers, and mortality in peripheral arterial disease: A substudy of the Iron (Fe) and

Atherosclerosis Study (FeAST) Trial. Journal of Vascular Surgery, 2010, Volume 51, Issue 6, 1498 – 1503.

5. Iqbal MP, Mehboobali N, Tareen AK, et al. Association of Body Iron Status with the Risk of Premature Acute Myocardial Infarction in a Pakistani Population. Kiechl S, ed. PLoS ONE. 2013;8(6):e67981.

6. Pourmoghaddas A, Sanei H, Garakyaraghi M, Esteki-Ghashghaei F, Gharaati M. The relation between body iron store and ferritin, and coronary artery disease. ARYA Atherosclerosis. 2014;10(1):32-36.

7. J. Hunnicutt, K. He, P. Xun. Dietary Iron Intake and Body Iron Stores Are Associated with Risk of Coronary Heart Disease in a Meta-Analysis of Prospective Cohort Studies. Journal of Nutrition, 2014; 144 (3): 359.

8. Lapice E., Masulli M., Vaccaro O. Iron deficiency and cardiovascular disease: An updated review of the evidence. Curr. Atheroscler. Rep. 2013;15:358.

9. Institute of Medicine. Food and Nutrition Board. Dietary Reference Intakes : a Report of the Panel on Micronutrients. Washington, DC: National Academy Press; 2001.

43. JUNK (FAST) FOOD

Introduction

Diet plays a crucial role in the development and prevention of cardiovascular disease.[1] The United States Department of Agriculture (USDA) describes fast food as "food purchased in self-service or carry-out eating places without wait service". It is mass produced and is prepared and served quickly. It is however caloric dense and is rich in refined sugars, sodium and saturated fats, including trans fats– dietary components that are detrimental for the cardiovascular health. Fast foods are usually short on cardiovascular friendly fiber, fruits and vegetables. Despite the health hazards, junk foods continue to grow in popularity.

Scientific Evidence

- There is a higher risk of dying from coronary heart disease by 20 percent in people who eat fast food once a week, when compared to people who avoid fast food. The risk increases by 50%, for people eating fast food two-three times each week and climbs to nearly 80 percent more, for people who consume fast food items four or more times each week.[2]
- Fast food is high in sodium [3] and for several years this content in fast foods has been on an increase. High sodium intake is a major cause of hypertension, and cardiovascular disease.
- Fast-food consumption results in weight gain and insulin resistance, factors that increases the risk of obesity and type 2 diabetes.[4] Fast food consumption has also been directly linked to an increased the incidence of type 2 diabetes.[5] Diabetes is a major risk factor for cardiovascular disease.
- Fast food is generally caloric dense, carries a high glycemic load and is served in large portions. There is a strong association between fast food consumption and obesity.[6]
- Fast food is high in saturated fat and trans-fatty acids, fats harmful to the cardiovascular system.[7]
- Fast foods are also rich in processed meats (like hot dogs). Processed meat consumption increases cardiovascular disease.[8]
- Fast food is also low in fiber, fruits and vegetables – and this is associated with a higher incidence of cardiovascular disease.

Conclusion

Fast foods are detrimental to the cardiovascular system. They encourage obesity, diabetes and hypertension – major cardiovascular risk factors. The USDA advises, choosing more fruits and vegetables, as salads or on sandwiches and pizza. They advise ordering 100% fruit juice to drink, instead of soda. They suggest choosing regular-size burgers, burritos, and tacos, not deluxe-size, avoiding or splitting a small order of fries, and ordering grilled chicken, not fried. Avoiding extra cheese on a pizza and going easy on mayonnaise, tartar sauce, special sauces, sour cream, salad dressings, and butter is also advisable.[9]

Lifestyle Implications

Avoid fast food as much as possible. Home cooking is healthy, economical, and helps build a family bond.

References

1. Nettleton JA, Polak JF, Tracy R, Burke GL, Jacobs DR., Jr Dietary patterns and incident cardiovascular disease in the Multi-Ethnic Study of Atherosclerosis. Am J Clin Nutr. 2009;90:647– 654.

2. Andrew O. Odegaard, Woon Puay Koh, Jian-Min Yuan, Myron D. Gross, and Mark A. Pereira. Western-Style Fast Food Intake and Cardio-Metabolic Risk in an Eastern Country. *Circulation*, July 2, 2012.

3. Cheng TO. Effects of fast foods, rising blood pressure and increasing serum cholesterol on cardiovascular disease in China. Am J Cardiol. 2006;97:1676–1678.

4. Pereira MA, Kartashov AI, Ebbeling CB, Van Horn L, Slattery ML, Jacobs DR, Jr, Ludwig DS. Fast-food habits, weight gain, and insulin resistance (the CARDIA study): 15-year prospective analysis. Lancet. 2005;365:36–42.

5. Odegaard AO, Koh WP, Butler LM, Duval S, Gross MD, Yu MC, Yuan JM, Pereira MA. Dietary patterns and incident type 2 diabetes in Chinese men and women: the Singapore Chinese Health Study. Diabetes Care. 2011;34:880– 885.

6. Rosenheck R. Fast food consumption and increased caloric intake: a systematic review of a trajectory towards weight gain and obesity risk. Obes Rev. 2008 Nov;9(6):535-47.

7. Mozaffarian D, Willett WC. Trans fatty acids and cardiovascular risk: a unique cardiometabolic imprint? Curr Atheroscler Rep. 2007 Dec;9(6):486-93.

8. Micha R, Wallace SK, Mozaffarian D. Red and processed meat consumption and risk of incident coronary heart disease, stroke, and

diabetes mellitus: a systematic review and meta-analysis. Circulation. 2010;121:2271–2283.

9. https://www.fns.usda.gov/sites/default/files/Nibbles_Newsletter_11.pdf.

44. LAUGHTER

Introduction

Laughter, a positive emotion, is ubiquitous in the human population. Smiling and laughter develop during infancy in the humans.[1] Smiling develops during the first 5 weeks of extrauterine life, while laughter emerges around the fourth month of life. These early human emotions play a significant role in defining the infant mother relationship. Laughter has significant physiological, psychological, social and spiritual benefits. Emerging data also substantiates the role of humor and mirthful laughter in beneficially modulating health, including cardiovascular health.[2]

Scientific Evidence

- Laughter reduces stress. Anticipatory anxiety is lower in people with the highest sense of humor. Humor and laughter also help reduce stress and anxiety in gravely sick patients.[3] Laughter therapy is beneficial in patients with depression.[4] Stress related cardiovascular damaging hormones such as cortisol, growth hormone and plasma dopamine, show a decrease after watching humorous movies.[5]

- Mirthful laughter is associated with short term 'aerobic exercise' like effects, as evidenced by muscle contractions, fast and sporadic deep breathing, increased heart-rate and improved oxygen consumption.[6] Controlled studies in healthy students have demonstrated that laughter is associated with improved heart function, as evidenced by significant increases in stroke volume and cardiac output. Laughter also helps motivate the elderly to participate in physical activity and to adhere to exercise programs.[7]

- Blood pressure may initially increase following a bout of laughter, but this is followed by a decrease. In a study involving 200 individuals involved in a regular practice of mirthful laughter, there was a 6.18 mm/Hg reduction in systolic blood pressure and a 3.82 mm/Hg reduction in diastolic blood pressure.[8] A reduction in blood pressure, as noted in this study, should translate into significant reductions in major cardiovascular events.

- Positive emotions like laughter improve the endothelial (inner lining of the blood vessels) function.[9] When compared to mental stress, mirthful laughter increases the diameter of the blood vessels and increases blood flow, while the former reduces it. Blood vessels constrict by as much as 30% to 50% on watching the stressful opening scene of 'Saving Private Ryan'. The reverse – an improvement in vessel diameter occurs in subjects on watching comedies such as 'There's something about Mary', 'Shallow Hall' and 'Kingpin'.[10] This positive endothelial benefit is helpful in preventing atherogenic vascular disease.

Conclusion

Laughter is a healthy emotion. It is also a universal bonding language. The beneficial health effects of social laughter, and mirthful laughter have been well studied and documented. Many of these effects positively improve cardiovascular risk factors and may help reduce cardiovascular disease and mortality.

Lifestyle Implications

Laughing is a serious matter, when it comes to a better cardiovascular health.

References

1. Sroufe LA, Waters E. The ontogenesis of smiling and laughter: a perspective on the organization of development in infancy. Psychol Rev. 1976, 83(3), 173-89.
2. Hayashi K, Kawachi I, Ohira T, Kondo K, Shirai K, Kondo N. Laughter is the Best Medicine? A Cross-Sectional Study of Cardiovascular Disease Among Older Japanese Adults. Journal of Epidemiology. 2016;26(10):546-552.
3. Leiber DB. Laughter and humor in critical care. Dimens Crit Care Nurs. 1976, 5, 162-70.
4. Shahidi M, Mojtahed A, Modabbernia A, Mojtahed M, Shafiabady A, Delavar A, Honari H. Laughter yoga versus group exercise program in elderly depressed women: a randomized controlled trial. Int J Geriatr Psychiatry, 2011, 26(3), 322-7.
5. Berk LS, Tan SA, Fry WF, Napier BJ, Lee JW, Hubbard RW, Lewis JE, Eby WC. Neuroendocrine and stress hormone changes during mirthful laughter. Am J Med Sci. 1989, 298(6), 390-6.
6. Fry W. The respiratory components of mirthful laughter. J Biol Psychol. 1977, 19, 39-50.
7. Hirosaki M, Ohira T, Kajiura M, Kiyama M, Kitamura A, Sato S, Iso H. Effects of a laughter and exercise program on physiological and

psychological health among communitydwelling elderly in Japan: randomized controlled trial. Geriatr Gerontol Int. 2013, 13(1), 152-60.

8. Chaya MS, Kataria M, Nagendra R, et al. American Society of Hypertension 2008 Annual Meeting; May 14, 2008; New Orleans, LA.

9. Miller M, Fry WF. The effect of mirthful laughter on the human cardiovascular system. Med Hypotheses, 2009, 73(5), 636-9.

10. Miller et al. Data presented at the European Society of Cardiology (ESC) Congress, 2011.

45. MAGNESIUM

Introduction

Magnesium (Mg) is the fourth most abundant mineral in the human body. It is estimated that 99% of total body Mg is located in bone, muscles and non-muscular soft tissue. Its role has been implicated in adenosine triphosphate metabolism, ribonucleic acid and deoxyribonucleic acid synthesis, protein producton and a multitude of crucial enzymatic reactions. It helps regulate muscular contraction, blood pressure, glucose metabolism insulin sensitivity, cardiac excitability, vasomotor tone and nerve transmission and neuromuscular conduction. Low levels of Mg have been associated with a number of chronic and inflammatory diseases, such as Alzheimer's disease, asthma, attention deficit hyperactivity disorder, eclampsia, type-2 diabetes mellitus, migraine headaches, depression, kidney stones and osteoporosis.[1] Its deficiency has also been implicated in several cardiovascular diseases.[2] Hypomagnesemia has been linked to an increase cardiovascular and all-cause mortality.[3]

Scientific Evidence

- Researchers studied 4,203 patients for a median duration of 10.1 years. Patients with low Mg levels were found to have a higher risk of coronary artery disease while those with high Mg levels had a reduced incidence of cardiovascular diseases and mortality.[3] This inverse association between Mg levels and coronary artery disease has been noted, both in women and men, in several other studies. Mg deficiency exacerbates the pathogenic atherosclerosis which invariably leads to ischemic heart disease.

- Similarly, an inverse relationship has been documented with Mg levels and stroke. In a meta-analysis of seven prospective studies, with 241,378 participants and 6,477 cases of stroke, Larrson and his associate found that low magnesium levels were associated with a higher incidence of ischemic stroke.[4] Mg reduces several risk factors for stroke including hypertension, diabetes mellitus and atrial fibrillation. Mg supplementation or a diet rich in Mg has also been effective in reducing the incidence of ischemic stroke.

- Low Mg levels may play a role in the development of several life-threatening ventricular arrhythmias and may increase the risk of sudden death.[5]
- Low levels of Mg have also been associated with hypertension, diabetes mellitus and the metabolic syndrome – all risk factors for the development of coronary heart disease.[6]

Conclusion

Mg plays an important role in human health and disease. Mg deficiency is inversely linked to cardiovascular disease and mortality. Mg intake remains low in the United States. According to the NHANES 2005–2006 survey, almost one half of all American adults have an inadequate nutritional intake of this mineral.[7] The recommended daily allowance for Mg in adults is 400 mg/day in men and 300-310 mg in women.[8] Daily requirements are higher in athletes, during pregnancy and lactation, and following a debilitating illness. Foods rich in Mg include dark leafy greens like spinach, nuts like almonds, seeds especially pumpkin seeds, fish, black beans, whole grains, avocados, yogurt or kefir, bananas, figs, dried fruit, and dark chocolate.

Lifestyle Implications

Magnesium levels are not routinely tested during a medical exam. With almost one half of all American adults not getting enough magnesium in their diet, and given the significance of its role in proper functioning of the body, it behooves one to eat foods rich in magnesium, especially dark leafy greens and seeds.

References

1. Song, Y.; Ridker, P.M.; Manson, J.E.; Cook, N.R.; Buring, J.E.; Liu, S. Magnesium intake, C-reactive protein, and the prevalence of metabolic syndrome in middle-aged and older U.S. Women. Diabetes Care 2005, 28, 1438–1444.

2. Qu X, Jin F, Hao Y, et al. Magnesium and the Risk of Cardiovascular Events: A Meta-Analysis of Prospective Cohort Studies. Malaga G, ed. PLoS ONE. 2013; 8(3): e57720.

3. Reffelmann T, Ittermann T, Dörr M, Völzke H, Reinthaler M, Petersmann A, Felix SB. Low serum magnesium concentrations predict cardiovascular and all-cause mortality. Atherosclerosis. 2011 Nov;219(1):280-4.

4. Larsson SC, Orsini N, Wolk A. Dietary magnesium intake and risk of stroke: A meta-analysis of prospective studies. Am J Clin Nutr. 2012; 95:362–366.

5. Del Gobbo LC, Song Y, Poirier P, Dewailly E, Elin RJ, Egeland GM. Low serum magnesium concentrations are associated with a high prevalence of premature ventricular complexes in obese adults with type 2 diabetes. Cardiovascular Diabetology. 2012;11:23.

6. Barbagallo M, Dominguez LJ. Magnesium and type 2 diabetes. World Journal of Diabetes. 2015;6(10):1152-1157.

7. CDC: Centers for Disease Control and Prevention. National Health and Nutrition Examination Survey. Available online: http://www.ars.usda.gov/SP2UserFiles/Place/80400530/pdf/0506/usual_nutrient_intake_vitD_ca_phos_mg_2005-06.pdf

8. IOM: Institute of Medicine, Food and Nutrition Board. Dietary Reference Intakes: Calcium, Phosphorus, Magnesium, Vitamin D and Fluoride. Washington, DC: National Academy Press, 1997.

46. MARGARINE

Introduction

Margarine is made from plant based oils such as canola oil, palm fruit oil and soybean oil. It was developed as a substitute for butter and is commonly used as a spread, for baking, and in cooking. Butter is made from animal fat while margarine is made from vegetable oils. However, hard margarine is high in trans-fat, which has been determined to be heart unhealthy. One tablespoon of stick margarine contains 1.5 to 25 grams of trans fats while light margarine and margarine with phytosterols contain no trans fats. Trans fats raise the bad low-density lipoprotein cholesterol and lower the good high-density lipoprotein cholesterol. Butter is rich in saturated fats, which also raise low-density lipoprotein cholesterol, but less than trans fats, and butter does not affect high-density lipoprotein cholesterol.

Scientific Evidence

- The role of dietary cholesterol in the pathogenesis of atherosclerosis and coronary artery disease has been well recognized.[1] Many subsequent studies revealed that intake of foods rich in trans fats resulted in a much higher risk of coronary heart disease.

- Investigators studied dietary data from 85,095 female participants in the Nurses' Health Study. They were all without coronary heart disease, stroke, diabetes, or high cholesterol levels on entry. During 8 years of follow-up, this population registered 431 cases of new coronary heart disease, both non-fatal and fatal. Researchers found that a high intake of trans fat foods such as margarine, cookies, cake, and white bread, was significantly associated with a higher risk of coronary heart disease.[2]

- In a prospective study of 667 men enrolled in the Zutphen Elderly Study, aged 64-84 years and free of coronary heart disease at baseline, researchers found that a high intake of trans fatty acids was associated with an increased risk of coronary heart disease.[3]

- Trans fats raise the 'bad' low-density lipoprotein cholesterol levels, when substituted for polyunsaturated fatty acids or carbohydrates. They also lower the levels of the 'good' high-density lipoprotein cholesterol, when substituted for unsaturated or saturated fatty acids.[4]

- Trans fatty acids increase inflammation, which can trigger or accelerate atherosclerosis.[5] There is also a detrimental effect on the endothelial function.[6]
- The US Food and Drug Administration (FDA) initially warned the public about the dangers of trans fat acids,[7] and has finally decided to ban these fats from human food.[8]

Conclusion

Margarine was developed as a substitute for butter. However, over the past few decades, several studies have shown that stick margarine is high in trans fats, the latter being atherogenic. Soft margarine appears to be safe. Given the strong evidence confirming the detrimental cardiovascular effects of trans fats, the FDA has issued an announcement banning these fats from human food.

Lifestyle Implications

Skip stick margarines as they are high in the heart unhealthy trans fat. Both butter and soft margarines are high in saturated fats, but may be used in moderation. Ideally, consider using olive oil as a spread on bread.

References

1. Keys A. Diet and the epidemiology of coronary heart disease. J. Am. Med. Assoc. 1957;164:1912–1919.
2. Willett WC, Stampfer MJ, Manson JE, Colditz GA, Speizer FE, Rosner BA, Sampson LA, Hennekens CH. Intake of trans fatty acids and risk of coronary heart disease among women. Lancet. 1993; 341: 581–585.
3. Oomen CM, Ocke MC, Feskens EJ, van Erp-Baart MA, Kok FJ, Kromhout D. Association between trans fatty acid intake and 10-year risk of coronary heart disease in the Zutphen Elderly Study: a prospective population-based study. Lancet. 2001; 357: 746–751.
4. Mensink RP, Zock PL, Kester AD, Katan MB. Effects of dietary fatty acids and carbohydrates on the ratio of serum total to HDL cholesterol and on serum lipids and apolipoproteins: a meta-analysis of 60 controlled trials. Am J Clin Nutr. 2003; 77: 1146–1155.
5. Baer DJ, Judd JT, Clevidence BA, Tracy RP. Dietary fatty acids affect plasma markers of inflammation in healthy men fed controlled diets: a randomized crossover study. Am J Clin Nutr. 2004; 79:969-973.
6. de Roos NM, Bots ML, Katan MB. Replacement of dietary saturated fatty acids by trans fatty acids lowers serum HDL cholesterol and impairs

endothelial function in healthy men and women. Arterioscler Thromb Vasc Biol. 2001; 21:1233-1237.

7. FDA1: http://www.fda.gov/oc/initiatives/transfat/.

8. FDA2: https://www.fda.gov/newsevents/newsroom/pressannouncements/ucm451237.htm.

47. MARRIAGE

Introduction

Marriage is a legally or a formally recognized union of two people as partners in a personal relationship. Married people have better general health than the unmarried,[1] They also have a better cardiovascular health and experience better outcomes following a heart attack.[2] They live longer than unmarried men and women.[3] The quality of marriage also matters - happily married women have better health than those that are unhappy. Married older adults with a social network exhibit a lesser degree of decline in their general health. Unfortunately, a large number of adults are single. According to the United States Census in 2014, there were 39,833,000 single adults, 50 years of age and older, living in the United States.[4] The majority of these older singles do not date and continue to remain single. This group is at an increased risk of poor health, including cardiovascular disease and early death.

Scientific Evidence

- Unmarried men have an increased risk of mortality when compared with married men.[5] Unmarried women also have an increased risk of early mortality.[6]
- Data from Scotland showed that separated or divorced women appeared to be protected and did not die early when compared to other unmarried women or men.[7]
- In a recent large study, researchers reviewed the records of over 3.5 million people. Their ages ranged from 21 to 102 years old. In this group, 69.1 percent (2.4 million) were married, 13 percent (477,577) were widowed, 8.3 percent (292,670) were single and 9 percent (319,321) were divorced. The data showed that marital status was independently associated with cardiovascular disease. Married people had 5% less vascular disease, 8% less abdominal aortic aneurysm, 9% less cerebrovascular disease and 19% less peripheral arterial disease. Widowers had a 7% higher odds of coronary artery disease.[8]
- A major factor responsible for the higher incidence of cardiovascular disease in some of these adults may be related to loneliness and social isolation. In meta-analysis of 16 longitudinal

datasets, poor social relationships increased the likelihood of coronary heart disease by 29% and stroke by 32%. Similar results have been reported from other studies.[9]

- Carotid intima media thickness is a surrogate for cardiovascular disease. A recent meta-analysis reported a 17% increase in the risk of myocardial infarction and stroke with an increase of only 0.1 mm in the common carotid intima media thickness, during a 4-year follow-up.[10] Negative marital interactions with high levels of hostility and low levels of warmth are associated with increased carotid artery intima thickening. These individuals have an 8.5% increased risk for myocardial infarction and stroke than those with positive marital interactions.

- An unhappy marriage is stressful and tends to cause depression. Depression increases the risk of cardiovascular diseases and death.

Conclusion

Marriage is health protective. Married men and women have less cardiovascular diseases, and lower mortality. Never married men and women and divorced men are at a higher risk of early mortality. However, marriage has to be happy and stable - troubled marriages are also associated with negative health consequences, especially in women

Lifestyle Implications

Get married, stay happy in your marriage, and you will live longer and healthier.

References

1. Kiecolt-Glaser JK, Newton TL. Marriage and health: His and hers. Psychological Bulletin. 2001;127:472–503.
2. Zhang Zhenmei, Hayward Mark D. Gender, the Marital Life Course, and Cardiovascular Health in Late Midlife. Journal of Marriage and Family. 2006;68:639–657.
3. Rendall MS, Weden MM, Favreault MM, et al. The protective effect of marriage for survival: a review and update. Demography. 2011 May;48(2):481-506.
4. United States Census Bureau. Families and Living Arrangements: America's Families and Living Arrangements: 2014: Adults. Table A1: Marital status of people 15 years and over, by age, sex, personal earnings, race, and Hispanic origin. 2014. https://www.census.gov/hhes/families/data/cps2014A.html.
5. Ben-Shlomo, Smith, Shipley, & Marmot, 1993); Ben-Shlomo Y, Smith GD, Shipley M, Marmot MG. Magnitude and causes of mortality

differences between married and unmarried men. Journal of Epidemiology and Community Health. 1993;47:200–205.

6. Cheung YB. Marital status and mortality in British women: A longitudinal study. International Journal of Epidemiology. 2000;29:93–99.

7. Molloy, Stamatakis, Randall, & Hamer, et al. Marital status, gender and cardiovascular mortality: Behavioural, psychological distress and metabolic explanations. Social Science & Medicine. 2009;69:223–228.

8. http://www.acc.org/about-acc/press-releases/2014/03/28/09/55/alviar-marital-status.

9. Julianne Holt-Lunstad, Timothy B. Smith, Mark Baker, Tyler Harris, David Stephenson. Loneliness and Social Isolation as Risk Factors for Mortality. Perspectives on Psychological Science.Vol 10, Issue 2, pp. 227 – 237

10. van den Oord SCH, Sijbrands EJG, ten Kate GL, van Klaveren D, van Domburg RT, van der Steen AFW, et al. Carotid intima-media thickness for cardiovascular risk assessment: systematic review and meta-analysis. Atherosclerosis. 2013;228:1–11.

48. MASSAGE

Introduction

Massage is commonly enjoyed as a relaxing activity during vacations. It is often used to reduce stress in the working population. Massage therapy is also used for several specific medical conditions, to promote healing.[1] Massage helps reduce pain and promote sleep. It also reduces blood pressure and heart rate, and improves immune function.[2,3] Its usefulness as a therapeutic modality to reduce blood pressure, respiratory rate, psychologic distress, and pain has been used in patients with cardiovascular diseases and in those undergoing cardiovascular procedures.[4]

Scientific Evidence

- In a study 263 volunteers, deep tissue massage of 45-60 minutes resulted in an average systolic pressure reduction of 10.4 mm Hg, and a diastolic pressure reduction of 5.3 mm. Average heart rate was reduced by 10.8 beats per minute.[5]
- In another study of 35 volunteers, 60 minutes following a full body massage, there was a reduction in both systolic and diastolic blood pressures.[6]
- Massage therapy helps a person reduces anxiety and relax. This may be beneficial for the cardiovascular system.[7] Reduction in anxiety following massage therapy has been documented in 64 patients with congestive heart failure.[8] In this study, back massage for 3 consecutive days, resulted in reduction in both systolic and diastolic blood pressure. The heart rate and breathing rates were also reduced. Their oxygen saturation levels in the blood were also significantly increased.
- In a study of 152 patients who had undergone cardiac surgery, a 20-minute massage significantly reduced the pain, anxiety, and muscular tension in these patients.[9]

Conclusion

Massage therapy is relaxing. It helps reduce anxiety. Blood pressure is reduced – though temporarily. Its use has been beneficial in patients with congestive heart failure and post cardiac surgery. Massage therapy is generally very safe – minor adverse effects have rarely been noted and include bruising, headache, and fatigue.[10,11] The majority of these adverse effects were associated with exotic types of manual massage or massage delivered by lay persons.[12]

Lifestyle Implications

Massage therapy is a good way to relax and reduce anxiety. It may help your cardiovascular system too. Enjoy an occasional full body massage.

References

1. Harris M. Richards KC. The physiological and psychological effects of slow-stroke back massage and hand massage on relaxation in older people. J Clin Nurs. 2010;19:917–926.
2. Richards KC. Effect of a back massage and relaxation intervention on sleep in critically ill patients. Am J Crit Care. 1998;7:288–299.
3. Goodfellow LM. The effects of therapeutic back massage on psychophysiologic variables and immune function in spouses of patients with cancer. Nurs Res. 2003;52:318–328.
4. McNamara ME. Burnham DC. Smith C. Carroll DL. The effects of back massage before diagnostic cardiac catheterization. Altern Ther Health Med. 2003;9:50–57.
5. Kaye AD, Kaye AJ, Swinford J, Baluch A, Bawcom BA, Lambert TJ, Hoover JM The effect of deep-tissue massage therapy on blood pressure and heart rate. J Altern Complement Med. 2008 Mar;14(2):125-8.
6. Sefton JM, Yarar C, Berry JW. Massage Therapy Produces Short-term Improvements in Balance, Neurological, and Cardiovascular Measures in Older Persons. International Journal of Therapeutic Massage & Bodywork. 2012;5(3):16-27.
7. Hatayama T, Kitamura S, Tamura C, et al. The facial massage reduced anxiety and negative mood status, and increased sympathetic nervous activity. Biomed Res. 2008;29(6):317–320.
8. Chen W-L, Liu G-J, Yeh S-H, Chiang M-C, Fu M-Y, Hsieh Y-K. Effect of Back Massage Intervention on Anxiety, Comfort, and Physiologic Responses in Patients with Congestive Heart Failure. Journal of Alternative and Complementary Medicine. 2013;19(5):464-470.
9. Braun LA, Stanguts C, Casanelia L, Spitzer O, Paul E, Vardaxis NJ, Rosenfeldt F. Massage therapy for cardiac surgery patients--a randomized trial. J Thorac Cardiovasc Surg. 2012 Dec;144(6):1453-9, 1459.e1.
10. Melancon B. Miller LH. Massage therapy versus traditional therapy for low back pain relief. Holist Nurs Pract. 2005;19:116–121.
11. Cambron JA. Dexheimer J. Coe P. Swenson R. Side-effects of massage therapy: A cross-sectional of 100 clients. J Altern Complement Med. 2007;13:793–796.

12. Ernst E. The safety of massage therapy. Rheumatology. 2003;42:1101–1106.

49. MEDICAL DISEASES

Introduction

Most organ specific diseases or systemic maladies have detrimental effects on the cardiovascular system. Cardiovascular involvement results in an impaired health status and worsened mortality. Although this topic can fill a textbook, we are mentioning some common conditions, involving different systems of the body, that negatively impact the cardiovascular system.

Scientific Evidence

- **Pulmonary:** Chronic Obstructive Pulmonary Disease affects the heart, often leading to right heart failure (cor pulmonale). The latter is responsible for between 10% and 30% of heart failure admissions in the US. One study found that chronic obstructive pulmonary disease was responsible for 84% of right heart failure cases.[1]

- **Endocrine**: Diabetes is now considered an independent cardiovascular risk factor. It is a common disease. It is estimated that at least 10.3 million Americans have this disease and another 5.4 million continue to remain undiagnosed. Approximately 65% of all diabetic deaths are due to cardiovascular diseases, including heart attacks, heart failure and stroke.[2]

- **Nephrology:** Chronic kidney disease adversely impacts the cardiovascular system. In a cohort study of 433 patients starting renal replacement therapy, 14% had proven coronary artery disease and 19% had symptomatic angina, with 32% showing left ventricular dilatation; 74% showing left ventricular hypertrophy and 31% had clinical heart failure.[3]

- **Neurology:** Dysautonomia involves failure of the sympathetic or parasympathetic components of the autonomic nervous system. An overactive autonomic nervous system is sometimes seen in neurological diseases such as Alzhiemer's and Guillian-Barre Syndrome. It can lead to low blood pressure and cause orthostatic hypotension, while excessive sympathetic activity can lead to hypertension and a rapid pulse. Cardiopulmonary arrest may occur in these patients.[4]

- **Oncology**: Cancer is one of the largest contributors to the burden of chronic disease in the United States. Cancer and cardiovascular diseases share several risk factors, especially inflammation – the latter being a major risk factor for atherosclerosis. Cancer treatment-related cardiotoxicity is a major cause of treatment-associated morbidity and mortality in cancer survivors.[5]
- **Hematology**: Patients with sickle cell disease have a plethora of cardiac complications and almost 40% of deaths are sudden and unexpected due to cardiovascular causes. Systemic lupus erythematosus, an immune system disorder, causes inflammation of the blood vessels – vasculitis. Women with lupus have heart attacks and strokes at a rate that is 9 times more than that seen in the general population. Death from cardiovascular diseases is 17 times higher than the general population, in these patients.[6]
- **Psychiatric**: There is a high comorbidity between psychiatric disorders and cardiovascular disease. Depression is a strongly associated with the development of cardiovascular diseases, including the occurance of major cardiac events and cardiovascular mortality. Anxiety independently predicts sudden cardiac death in the general population. It also prognosticates increased future cardiac events in patients with cardiovascular diseases. There is an increased mortality, primarily from cardiovascular causes, in schizophrenia – and this is approximately two to three times higher than that seen in the general population.[7] Bipolar patients also exhibit twice the cardiovascular mortality compared to the general population.
- **Nutritional:** Nearly 70% of American adults are either overweight or obese. Obesity is associated with many cardiovascular risk factors including abnormal lipids, insulin resistance, increased inflammation and an increased tendency to form blood clots. It is estimated that 21 per cent of chronic heart disease worldwide is attributable to a body mass index above 21.

Conclusion

Many medical diseases affect the cardiovascular system. It is therefore important to get a regular physical exam and take care of any medical conditions one may have, to prevent or minimize their deleterious effects on the cardiovascular system.

Lifestyle Implications

Get an annual medical exam and follow your health care provider's instructions properly — especially if you have been diagnosed with an ailment.

References

1. MacNee W. Pathophysiology of cor pulmonale in chronic obstructive pulmonary disease: part one. Am J Respir Crit Care Med. 1994; 150: 833–852.
2. Geiss LS, Herman WH, Smith PJ, National Diabetes Data Group. Diabetes in America. Bethesda, Md: National Institutes of Health, National Institute of Diabetes and Digestive and Kidney Diseases; 1995:233–257.
3. Foley RN, Parfrey PS, Harnett JD, et al. Clinical and echocardiographic disease in patients starting end-stage renal disease therapy. Kidney Int. 1995;47:186.
4. Ninds: https://www.ninds.nih.gov/Disorders/All-Disorders/Dysautonomia-information-Page
5. Morris PG, Hudis CA. Trastuzumab-related cardiotoxicity following anthracycline- based adjuvant chemotherapy: how worried should we be? J Clin Oncol. 2010;28:3407–3410.
6. Lupus: http://resources.lupus.org/entry/preventive-cardiac-care.
7. Ringen PA, Engh JA, Birkenaes AB, et al. Increased Mortality in schizophrenia due to Cardiovascular Disease – A Non-Systematic Review of Epidemiology, Possible Causes, and Interventions. Frontiers in Psychiatry. 2014;5:137.

50. MEDITERRANEAN DIET

Introduction

People living in the olive growing regions of the Mediterranean basin follow a diet that is high in monounsaturated fats; wine intake at low to moderate levels; high consumption of vegetables, fruits, nuts, seeds, legumes, and grains; moderate consumption of milk and dairy products, mostly in the form of cheese; high intake of olive oil; more sourdough bread than pasta; low to moderate amounts of fish and poultry; eggs zero to four times a week and low consumption of red meat and meat products. This diet is low in saturated fat (< or = 7-8% of energy), with a high monounsaturated/saturated fats ratio and with total fats providing 25% to 35% of energy. The Mediterranean diet has been linked with several health benefits, including a decreased incidence of adult onset diabetes mellitus, reduced incidence of several cancers and less hip fractures. There is also a beneficial association noted with cardiovascular diseases.[1]

Scientific Evidence

- Studies indicate that the Mediterranean diet (MeD) may help prevent the development of hypertension, reduce both systolic and diastolic blood pressure, and help in its control.[2]
- Several studies have shown that MeD is good for diabetic patients, leading to a better glycemic control, higher rates of diabetes remission, delayed need for diabetes medication, reduction in cardiovascular risk factors and in improving the quality of life of these patients. Metabolic syndrome is a pre-diabetic state and MeD is associated with a 15% to 80% reduced risk of developing this syndrome. MeD, as compared with regular diets, may reduce glycated hemoglobin (HbA1c) levels by 0.30–0.47%.[3]
- Several facets of obesity are positively improved by MeD, especially a decrease in abdominal obesity. Several other studies have confirmed a similar inverse relationship between adherence to MeD and overweight/obesity.[4]
- MeD is associated with beneficial effects on the lipids as evidenced by decreased amount of oxidized low-density lipoprotein cholesterol levels. Virgin olive oil helps enhance the high-density lipoprotein cholesterol related atherosclerotic protection.[5]

- A host of studies on the primary prevention of cardiovascular disease show a statistically significant positive association between adherance to the MedDiet and reduction in the incidence of cardiovascular diseases. Addition of extra-virgin olive oil or mixed nuts to the MeD reduce the cardiovascular events by 30%. There was a coronary heart disease mortality reduction of 26% at 20 years and 22% reduction at 40 years in individuals with a higher adherence to the MeD in Italy.[6]

- Heart failure biomarkers improve with MeD as evidenced by a reduction in the N-terminal pro-brain natriuretic peptide. MeD is also associated with a lower risk of stroke. A beneficial effect has also been seen in patients with peripheral vascular disease.[7] The beneficial effects of MeD on cardiovascular risk factors and cardiovascular diseases results in reduced cardiovascular mortality.[8]

Conclusion

The evidence regarding MeD in increasing protection from cardiovascular diseases, is strong. MeD diet is primarily a plant based diet, with only low intakes of red meat. Its cardioprotective benefits accrue from its positive effects on lipid profile, endothelial function, vascular inflammation, and insulin resistance. With the increasing worldwide prevalence of cardiovascular disease, dietary incorporation and subsequent adherence to the MeD, can greatly help in curbing the number one killer in the world.

Lifestyle Implications

Incorporate Mediterranean diet, as much as possible, in your eating habits.

References

1. Rees K., Hartley L., Flowers N., et al. Mediterranean dietary pattern for the primary prevention of cardiovascular disease. Cochrane Database Syst. Rev. 2013;8.
2. Toledo E, Hu FB, Estruch R, Buil-Cosiales P, et al. Effect of the Mediterranean diet on blood pressure in the PREDIMED trial: results from a randomized controlled trial. BMC Med. 2013 Sep 19;11:207.
3. Esposito K, Maiorino MI, Bellastella G, et al. A journey into a Mediterranean diet and type 2 diabetes: a systematic review with meta-analyses. BMJ Open. 2015;5(8): e008222.
4. Lazarou C., Panagiotakos D.B., Matalas A.L. Physical activity mediates the protective effect of the Mediterranean diet on children's obesity status: The CYKIDS study. Nutrition. 2010;26:61–67.

5. Hernáez A, Castañer O, Elosua R, et al. Mediterranean diet improves high-density lipoprotein function in high-cardiovascular-risk individuals: A randomized controlled trial. Circulation 2017; 135:633-643.

6. Menotti A., Alberti-Fidanza A., Fidanza F. The association of the Mediterranean Adequacy Index with fatal coronary events in an Italian middle-aged male population followed for 40 years. Nutr. Metab. Cardiovasc. Dis. 2012;22:369.

7. Ruiz-Canela M, Estruch R, Corella D, et al. Association of Mediterranean diet with peripheral artery disease: the PREDIMED randomized trial. JAMA. 2014;311:415–417.

8. Tong TYN, Wareham NJ, Khaw K-T, Imamura F, Forouhi NG. Prospective association of the Mediterranean diet with cardiovascular disease incidence and mortality and its population impact in a non-Mediterranean population: the EPIC-Norfolk study. BMC Medicine. 2016;14:135.

51. MENTAL DISEASES

Introduction

Mental disorders are common – it is estimated that approximately 1 in 5 adults (18.5%) in the U.S. experiences a mental illness every year. The common diseases are anxiety (including posttraumatic stress disorder, obsessive-compulsive disorder and phobias), depression, bipolar disorders and schizophrenia. Mental disorders are more common in homeless people, prisoners and juvenile offenders. People with serious mental illnesses are at an increased risk of having chronic medical conditions.[1] Their lifespan is reduced by almost 25 years.[2] Mental illnesses also increase the risk of cardiovascular disease.

Scientific Evidence

- Anxiety independently predicts sudden cardiac death in the general population. It also prognosticates increased future cardiac events in patients with cardiovascular diseases, including mortality.[3] Patients with chronic anxiety suffer from elevated sympathetic nervous system activity, increased inflammation, and often hypertension – all increasing the risk of cardiovascular diseases.[4]

- Depression is a strong predictor for the development of cardiovascular diseases, including major cardiac events and cardiovascular mortality. People with depression increase their risk of cardiovascular disease by 1.6 to 1.8 times when compared to those without depression.[5] In patients with cardiovascular disease, depression also increases the risk by 1.8 to 2.6 times for a subsequent cardiovascular event or death.[6]

- There is an increased mortality rate, primarily from cardiovascular causes, in schizophrenia - approximately two to three times higher than in the general population.[7] A large Taiwanese study showed that the patients with schizophrenia suffered from a 1.26-fold higher risk of peripheral arterial disease than those without schizophrenia.[8] Patients with peripheral arterial disease are at a high risk of adverse cardiovascular events.

- Bipolar patients also have over 2 times the cardiovascular mortality than the general population.[9]

- Causes for the increased risk for cardiovascular diseases and events in patients with psychiatric problems are multifactorial and include excessive use of tobacco and alcohol, chronic stress, poor diet and lack of physical activity. They often suffer from metabolic diseases. Psychiatric medications can also lead to obesity, high cholesterol and diabetes. These patients are often hesitant in seeking help or communicating health issues with their health care provider.

Conclusion

Psychiatric illnesses are common. These patients also suffer from several medical co-morbidities. Cardiovascular events such as heart attacks and stroke are approximately twice as common in this population when compared to the general public. Patients with mental illness lose an average of 25 years of life. Causes are multifactorial.

Lifestyle Implications

If you feel depressed or suffer from uncontrollable anxiety – get psychiatric help. Proper treatment of a mental illness may help reduce your risk for cardiovascular disease.

References

1. Colton, C.W. & Manderscheid, R.W. (2006). Congruencies in Increased Mortality Rates, Years of Potential Life Lost, and Causes of Death Among Public Mental Health Clients in Eight States. Preventing Chronic Disease: Public Health Research, Practice and Policy, 3(2), 1–14. Retrieved from http://www.ncbi.nlm.nih.gov/pmc/articles/PMC1563
2. Alexandria et al, National Association of State Mental Health Program Directors Council. (2006). Morbidity and Mortality in People with Serious Mental Illness. Retrieved from http://www.nasmhpd.org/docs/publications/MDCd
3. Schulman J.K., Philip R. Muskin, and Peter A. Shapiro. Psychiatry and Cardiovascular Disease. Focus. Volume 3, Issue 2, April 2005, pp. 208-224.
4. Watkins LL, Koch GG, Sherwood A, et al. Association of Anxiety and Depression With All-Cause Mortality in Individuals With Coronary Heart Disease. Journal of the AHA: Cardiovascular and Cerebrovascular Disease. 013;2(2):e000068.
5. Nicholson A, Kuper H, Hemingway H. Depression as an aetiologic and prognostic factor in coronary heart disease: a meta-analysis of 6362 events among 146 538 participants in 54 observational studies. Eur. Heart J. 2006;27:2763–2774.

6. Barth J, Schumacher M, Herrmann-Lingen C. Depression as a risk factor for mortality in patients with coronary heart disease: a meta-analysis. Psychosom. Med. 2004;66:802–813.

7. Ringen PA, Engh JA, Birkenaes AB, Dieset I, Andreassen OA. Increased Mortality in Schizophrenia Due to Cardiovascular Disease – A Non-Systematic Review of Epidemiology, Possible Causes, and Interventions. Frontiers in Psychiatry. 2014;5:137.

8. Hsu W-Y, Lin C-L, Kao C-H. A Population-Based Cohort Study on Peripheral Arterial Disease in Patients with Schizophrenia. Pizzi C, ed. PLoS ONE. 2016;11(2): e0148759.

9. Crump C, Sundquist K, Winkleby MA, Sundquist J. Comorbidities and mortality in bipolar disorder: a Swedish national cohort study. JAMA Psychiatry (2013) 70:931–910.1001/jamapsychiatry.2013.1394.

52. MILK

Introduction

Milk is produced by mammals as the primary nutrition for thier infants. However, milk continues to be used as food in humans beyond infancy. It is estimated that 730 million tonnes of milk was produced in 2011 from 260 million dairy cows. Milk is high in saturated fat and has therefore been implicated as a possible risk factor in increasing the risk of ischemic heart disease, stroke, and total mortality. The U.S. Department of Agriculture and U.S. Department of Health and Human Services recommend only low-fat and fat-free milk and their products as part of a healthy diet to reduce the risk of cardiovascular diseases.[1] They recommend consumption of three glasses of fat-free or low-fat milk for adults and children 9 years of age and older per day. The scientific data on the relationship of whole milk with increased cardiovascular disease however is neither definite nor consistent.[2,3]

Scientific Evidence

- In a meta-analysis of 17 prospective studies (total of 611,430 participants, followed for 14-16 years and involving 2,283 cardio-vascular disease cases, and 4,391 coronary heart disease events (15,554 strokes, and 23,949 deaths), researchers found that milk intake was not associated with total mortality but may have an inverse relationship with the overall cardiovascular risk.[3]
- In another meta-analysis of 38 studies, data suggests that there is a small but worthwhile reduction in the risk of coronary heart disease and a reduction in all strokes and hemorrhagic stroke in subjects who drank the most milk.[2]
- Results from short-term intervention studies on cardiovascular disease biomarkers have indicated that a diet higher in whole milk increases both low-density lipoprotein cholesterol and high-density lipoprotein cholesterol, and does not alter the total cholesterol/high-density lipoprotein cholesterol ratio. They concluded that there was no association between the intake of milk fat and the risk of coronary heart disease and stroke.[4]
- Swedish researchers, in 2014, reported that higher milk consumption was associated with a doubling of mortality risk including cardiovascular disease mortality in women.[5]

- A recent meta-analysis data from 29 prospective cohort studies demonstrated neutral associations between dairy products, including milk, and cardiovascular and all-cause mortality.[6]

Conclusion

Animal milk (especially from cattle, sheep and goats) has been consumed by adult humans as far back as the Neolithic times. Milk has been considered bad for the cardiovascular system mainly due to its high content of saturated fat. However, most prospective cohort studies and meta-analyses have showed either no relationship or an inverse association (beneficial), between milk intake and the risk of cardiovascular disease and stroke.

Lifestyle Implications

Drink whole milk, if you want to, but watch your saturated fat intake – it should not exceed 10% of your total calories. Low fat or fat free milk is safe for the cardiovascular system.

References

1. U.S. Department of Agriculture and U.S. Department of Health and Human Services. Dietary guidelines for Americans, 2010. 7th ed. Washington, DC: U.S. Government Printing Office, 2010.
2. Elwood PC, Pickering JE, Givens DI, Gallacher JE. The consumption of milk and dairy foods and the incidence of vascular disease and diabetes: an overview of the evidence. Lipids. 2010;45:925–39
3. Soedamah-Muthu SS, Ding EL, Al-Delaimy WK, Hu FB, Engberink MF, Willett WC, Geleijnse JM. Milk and dairy consumption and incidence of cardiovascular diseases and all-cause mortality: dose-response meta-analysis of prospective cohort studies. Am J Clin Nutr. 2011;93:158–71.
4. Huth PJ, Park KM. Influence of Dairy Product and Milk Fat Consumption on Cardiovascular Disease Risk: A Review of the Evidence. Advances in Nutrition. 2012;3(3):266-285.
5. Michaelsson K, Wolk A, Langenskiold S, Basu S, Warensjo Lemming E, Melhus H, Byberg L. Milk intake and risk of mortality and fractures in women and men: cohort studies. BMJ. 2014;349: g6015.
6. Guo J, Astrup A, Lovegrove JA, Gijsbers L, Givens DI, Soedamah-Muthu SS. Milk and dairy consumption and risk of cardiovascular diseases and all-cause mortality: dose–response meta-analysis of prospective cohort studies. European Journal of Epidemiology. 2017;32(4):269-287.

53. MINDFULNESS

Introduction

Mindfulness is defined as "paying attention in a particular way: on purpose, in the present moment, and non-judgmentally".[1] It has been practiced and prescribed successfully for a reduction of anxiety, depression and stress. Besides neuro-psychological benefits, mindfulness also positively affects many physical ailments, including cardiovascular diseases.[2]

Scientific Evidence

- Mindfulness practice reduces blood pressure.[3] This has been shown in low income African Americans, breast cancer survivors, and prostate cancer patients. Small reductions have significant effects on major end points. A 5 mm/Hg systolic blood pressure reduction can decrease the risk for stroke by 34% and the risk for ischemic heart disease by 21%.[4]

- Mindfulness practice also helps diabetic patients. They notice a better sugar control, enhanced emotional well-being and an improved quality of life.[5]

- Mindfulness reduces neurogenic inflammation, and may play a role in reducing vascular inflammation.[6] Further studies are needed to better elucidate this association. Reduction in vascular inflammation helps reduce cardiovascular events.

- Mind body relaxation techniques appear to favorably ater the cholesterol levels. Studies on transcendental meditation patients have reported improvements in the lipid profile.[7] Similar responses are expected with mindfulness meditation.

- Mindfulness techniques also favorably affect lifestyle risk factors for cardiovascular disease such as smoking, alcoholism, obesity and physical inactivity.

- Mindfulness also reduces anxiety and depression in patients with hypertension.[8] It also has significant effects in reducing depression in non-hypertensives.[9] Treatment of depression itself reduces future cardiovascular events in otherwise healthy individuals and following a cardiovascular event. Mindfulness meditation can attenuate anxiety in both healthy patients and those with generalized anxiety disorder.[10] The favorable effects induced by mindfulness practice should help reduce the detrimental emotional burden in patients with cardiovascular diseases.

Conclusion

The mechanism behind the benefits of mindfulness meditation in cardiovascular diseases include a reduction in stress, anxiety and depression, and lowering of inflammation and oxidation There is also a positive modulation of the autonomic nervous system. Mindfulness also helps decrease several cardiovascular risk factors including smoking, inactivity, obesity, hypertension, diabetes mellitus, and excessive alcohol intake. Mindfulness is easy to learn and easy to incorporate into normal life.

Lifestyle Implications

Regular mindfulness practice will improve your emotional state and can also help reduce your risk for cardiovascular disease.

References

1. Kabat-Zinn, 2003; Kabat-Zinn J. (2003). Mindfulness-based interventions in context: past, present, and future. Clin. Psychol. Sci.Pract. 10, 144–156.
2. Indranill Basu Ray, Arthur R. Menezes, Pavan Malur, et al. Meditation and Coronary Heart Disease: A Review of the Current Clinical Evidence. Ochsner J. 2014 Winter; 14(4): 696–703.
3. Carlson LE, Speca M, Faris P, et al. One-year pre-post intervention follow-up of psychological, immune, endocrine and blood pressure outcomes of mindfulness-based stress reduction (MBSR) in breast and prostate cancer outpatients. Brain Behav Immun. 2007 Nov; 21(8):1038-49.
4. Law M, Wald N, Morris J. Lowering blood pressure to prevent myocardial infarction and stroke: a new preventive strategy. Health Technol Assess. 2003; 7(31):1-94.
5. Hartmann M, Kopf S, Kircher C, et al. Sustained effects of a mindfulness-based stress-reduction intervention in type 2 diabetic patients: design and first results of a randomized controlled trial (the Heidelberger Diabetes and Stress-study). Diabetes Care. 2012 May; 35(5):945-7.
6. William B. Malarkey, David Jarjoura, Maryanna Klatt, et al. Workplace based mindfulness practice and inflammation: A randomized trial. Brain Behav Immun. 2013 Jan; 27(1): 145–154.
7. Paul-Labrador M, Polk D, Dwyer JH, et al. Effects of a randomized controlled trial of transcendental meditation on components of the metabolic syndrome in subjects with coronary heart disease. Arch Intern Med. 2006, 166(11):1218-24.

8. Parswani MJ, Sharma MP, Iyengar S. Mindfulness-based stress reduction program in coronary heart disease: A randomized control trial. Int J Yoga. 2013 Jul; 6(2):111-7.

9. Clara Strauss, Kate Cavanagh, Annie Oliver, et al. Mindfulness-Based Interventions for People Diagnosed with a Current Episode of an Anxiety or Depressive Disorder: A Meta-Analysis of Randomised Controlled Trials. PLoS One. 2014; 9(4): e96110.

10. Zeidan F, Martucci KT, Kraft RA, McHaffie JG, Coghill RC. Neural correlates of mindfulness meditation-related anxiety relief. Social Cognitive and Affective Neuroscience. 2014;9(6):751-759.

54. MONEY: SOCIO-ECONOMIC STATUS

Introduction

Economic disadvantage has significant negative repercussions on the cardiovascular health of people, especially women. Prevalence, prospective, and retrospective cohort studies, have established an inverse relationship between a low socioeconomic status and cardiovascular risk factors and major cardiovascular events, including fatality. Patients on the lower end of the socioeconomic ladder (especially women), often lead a more sedentary lifestyle, smoke more, eat less fruits and vegetables, are obese, suffer from diabetes, and have chronic stress. They also tend to suffer from several other harmful risk factors for cardiovascular diseases.

Scientific Evidence

- In a study of 819 women, prospectively enrolled in the Women's Ischemia Syndrome Evaluation, researchers found that low socioeconomic factors were associated with an elevated risk of cardiovascular death or a heart attack. These participants included those with an annual household income <$20,000, 9th grade education, being African American, Hispanic, Asian, or American Indian, getting Medicaid, Medicare, or other public health insurance, unmarried, unemployed or employed part-time and/or working in a service job. Low income was the main predictor of cardiovascular death or heart attack in these patients.[1]

- In a record-linkage cohort study of 1.93 million people to examine the association between small-area socioeconomic deprivation and 12 cardiovascular diseases, researchers found that the impact of socioeconomic deprivation on increased cardiovascular disease was real, but is often absent in men and only seen in women.[2]

- In a study called the Swedish Surveys of Living Conditions, working conditions and wages were used to review the cardiovascular health of 6,405 people between 1996-1999, and a seperate data of 10,916 cardiovascular deaths for the period 1990-95. These studies revealed that those in the lowest income quartile had 3.6 times higher risk of getting cardiovascular disease and a 2.1 times higher risk of death from cardiovascular disease, when compared to those in the highest income quartile.[3]

- The causes of this association are multifactorial. People in the upper socioeconomic levels have healthier behaviors and lifestyles compared to people in the lower socioeconomic levels. The poorer group suffers from more diabetes and obesity. They also eat fewer fruits and vegetables. Other factors include poor access to health information and health services, chronic stress, increased smoking and a more sedentary lifestyle.[4]
- Development of cardiovascular disease by itself increases the risk of sliding into a lower socio-economic status.[5]

Conclusions

A higher socio-economic status translates into a better cardiovascular health and cardiovascular future, especially in women. People with lower income have poorer lifestyles and higher cardiovascular risk factors.

Lifestyle Implications

A lower socio-economic status puts you at a higher risk of serious cardiovascular events, especially if you are a female. If you fall in this group, you need to pay more attention to healthy cardiovascular lifestyles – eat more fruits and vegetables, exercise, do not smoke and monitor your blood pressure and blood sugar.

References

1. Shaw LJ, Bairey Merz CN, Bittner V, et al. Importance of Socioeconomic Status as a Predictor of Cardiovascular Outcome and Costs of Care in Women with Suspected Myocardial Ischemia. Results from the National Institutes of Health, National Heart, Lung and Blood Institute-Sponsored Women's Ischemia Syndrome Evaluation (WISE). Journal of Women's Health. 2008;17(7):1081-1092.
2. Pujades-Rodriguez M, Timmis A, Stogiannis D, et al. Socioeconomic Deprivation and the Incidence of 12 Cardiovascular Diseases in 1.9 Million Women and Men: Implications for Risk Prediction and Prevention. Woodward M, ed. PLoS ONE. 2014;9(8): e104671.
3. Toivanen S, Hemström O. Income differences in cardiovascular disease: is the contribution from work similar in prevalence versus mortality outcomes? Int J Behav Med. 2006;13(1):89-100.
4. J.P. Pierce et al., "Trends in Cigarette Smoking in the United States: Educational Differences Are Increasing," Journal of the American Medical Association 26, no. 1 (1989): 56–60.

5.   Callander EJ, Schofield DJ. The risk of falling into poverty after
      developing heart disease: a survival analysis. BMC Public Health.
      2016;16:570.

149

55. MUSIC

Introduction

Music is considered an art form and is deeply ingrained in many people's way of life. Besides pleasure, it also plays an important role in social activities like dancing, exercising, religious rituals, ceremonies such as graduation and marriage and many other cultural activities. It dates back several centuries according to historians. Recently, a flute (Divje Babe flute), carved from a cave bear femur, was found and is thought to be about 40,000 years old.[1] Music is also used as a complimentary therapy to promote health in several health ailments, such as reducing agitation in psychiatry patients,[2] relaxing patients in stressful situations,[3] and reducing pain, anxiety and distress in post-operative patients.[4] It is also helpful in reducing stress in patients with coronary heart disease.[5] Music can help slow the heart rate, lower blood pressure, reduce levels of stress hormones and inflammatory cytokines - all risk factors for coronary heart disease.

Scientific Evidence

- Researchers reviewed 26 trials, with1,369 participants, on the effects of music on several cardiac parameters in patients with coronary heart disease. They found that listening to music reduces heart rate, respiratory rate and systolic blood pressure. There was also a reduction in stress and anxiety and improved sleep.[3]
- In a study of 60 patients undergoing open heart surgery, relaxing music helped reduce postoperative pain.[6]
- A study of 60 stroke patients recruited between March 2004 and May 2006 from the Department of Neurology of the Helsinki University Central Hospital, cognitive recovery and prevention of negative mood was enhanced in the early post-stroke phase with music.[7]
- Slow or meditative music can also induce relaxation, particularly during the musical pauses.[8]
- In cardiac rehabilitation, music increases the time of physical activity undertaken and helps in exercise adherence.[9]

- Meditative or slow classical music also helps reduce levels of stress hormones, thrombotic activity and inflammatory cytokines – all risk factors for coronary heart disease.[10]

Conclusions

Not all music is created equal. Slow and meditative music has been found to be therapeutic. Studies in heart disease patients validate the stress relieving, and harmful biomarker decreasing, effects of music. Music improves the quality of life of patients. The reductions in blood pressure with music therapy, although small, may have significant long-term effects. It is estimated that a small reduction of 5 mmHg in systolic blood pressure, would result in 7 % reduction in all-cause mortality, 9 % reduction in coronary heart disease related mortality and 14 % reduction in stroke-related mortality. Although no specific objective studies are reported in the scientific literature substantiating the long-term benefits of music on the cardiovascular system, these studies do suggest that music is good for the heart and the blood vessels.

Lifestyle Implications

Music is good for your heart – especially if it is slow and meditative. It helps reduce stress, anxiety and depression.

References

1. https://en.wikipedia.org/wiki/Music
2. Ridder HMO, Stige B, Qvale LG, Gold C. Individual music therapy for agitation in dementia: an exploratory randomized controlled trial. Aging Ment Health. 2013;17(6):67–678.
3. Bradt J, Dileo C, Shim M. Music interventions for preoperative anxiety. Cochrane Database Syst Rev. 2013 Jun 6; (6):CD006908.
4. Van der Heijden MJE, Oliai Araghi S, van Dijk M, Jeekel J, Hunink MGM. The Effects of Perioperative Music Interventions in Pediatric Surgery: A Systematic Review and Meta-Analysis of Randomized Controlled Trials. Laks J, ed. PLoS ONE. 2015;10(8): e0133608.
5. Bradt J, Dileo C, Potvin N. Music for stress and anxiety reduction in coronary heart disease patients. Cochrane Database Syst Rev. 2013 Dec 28;(12):CD006577.
6. Mirbagher Ajorpaz N, Mohammadi A, Najaran H, Khazaei S. Effect of Music on Postoperative Pain in Patients Under Open Heart Surgery. Nursing and Midwifery Studies. 2014;3(3): e20213.

7. Teppo Sa«rka«mo, Mari Tervaniemi, Sari Laitinen et al. Music listening enhances cognitive recovery and mood after middle cerebral artery stroke. Brain (2008), 131, 866 – 876.

8. Bernardi L, Porta C, Sleight P. Cardiovascular, cerebrovascular, and respiratory changes induced by different types of music in musicians and non-musicians: the importance of silence. Heart. 2006;92(4):445-452.

9. Alter DA, O'Sullivan M, Oh PI, et al. Synchronized personalized music audio-playlists to improve adherence to physical activity among patients participating in a structured exercise program: a proof-of-principle feasibility study. Sports Medicine - Open. 2015;1:23.

10. Möckel M, Röcker L, Störk T, et al. Immediate physiological responses of healthy volunteers to different types of music: cardiovascular, hormonal and mental changes. Eur J Appl Physiol Occup Physiol. 1994; 68(6):451-9.

56. NEGATIVITY

Introduction

Persistent negative emotions are believed to increase the risk for atherosclerosis and cardiovascular disease by raising the levels of inflammation causing chemicals in the body and inducing several harmful neuro-hormonal changes. Negative emotions include anger, depression, despair, doubt, envy, fear, frustration, grief, guilt, hate, hostility, jealousy, sadness, shame, etc. The ability to accept and cope with negative emotions is psychologically better than avoidance or suppression – the latter may lead to clinical psychopathology, including anxiety and depression. Acceptance and coping with negativity is considered preventive in the development of this psychopathology, while avoidance or suppression is dangerous not only to the psyche, but also the physical body. Several scientific studies have demonstrated that negative emotions are associated with poor health,[1] including increased cardiovascular disease,[2] and higher mortality.[3] The harmful cardiovascular response is mediated via the autonomic nervous system, manifesting as an increased sympathetic tone - experimentally documented as a lower heart rate variability.

Scientific Evidence

- Western cultures have shown that negative emotions predict higher levels of pro-inflammatory biomarkers,[4] specifically Interleukin-6. Increased inflammation leads to enhanced atherosclerosis and eventually cardiovascular disease.[5]
- Many negative emotions, especially depression, have been shown to be independently associated with a higher risk of cardiovascular disease and cardiovascular mortality. In a meta-analysis of sixteen studies, depressed patients had a 39% increased risk of cardiovascular mortality.[6]
- Negative marital interactions with high levels of hostility and low levels of warmth induce an approximately 8.5% increased risk for myocardial infarction and stroke – when compared to those in a positive marital relationship.[7]
- Carotid intima media thickness is a surrogate marker for cardiovascular disease and a recent meta-analysis reported a 17%

increase in the risk of myocardial infarction and stroke with only a 0.1 mm difference (increase) in common carotid carotid intima media thickness during a 4 years of follow-up.[8]

Conclusions

Negative emotions and positive emotions co-exist in nature and are often experienced in concert. The ability to experience and competently handle these has been associated with improved physical health.[9] Inability to accept them or an attempt to suppress them is associated with increased systemic inflammation, stimulation of the sympathetic nervous system, enhanced atherosclerosis and premature cardiovascular disease.

Lifestyle Implications

People usually prefer positive emotions and tend to avoid negative emotions. However, in life, these two commonly coexist. Negative emotions should be accepted and not avoided or suppressed. This will help you to be more emotionally stable. Overall, stay positive, stay optimistic, and laugh – life is short. These lifestyle practices will help improve your long-term psychological and physical well-being – and help reduce future incidence of cardiovascular diseases.

References

1. Penninx BWJH, Guralnik JM, Pahor M, Ferrucci L, Cerhan JR, Wallace RB, Havlik RJ. Chronically depressed mood and cancer risk in older persons. J Natl Cancer Inst. 1998;90:1888–1893.
2. Kubzansky LD, Kawachi I. Going to the heart of the matter: do negative emotions cause coronary heart disease? J Psychosom Res. 2000;48:323–337.
3. Pinquart M, Duberstein PR. Depression and cancer mortality: a meta-analysis. Psychol Med. 2010;40:1979–1810.
4. Miyamoto Y, Boylan JM, Coe CL, et al. Negative Emotions Predict Elevated Interleukin-6 in the United States but not in Japan. Brain, behavior, and immunity. 2013; 34:10.1016/j. bbi.2013.07.173.
5. Ridker PM, Rifai N, Stampfer MJ, Hennekens CH. Plasma concentration of interleukin-6 and the risk of future myocardial infarction among apparently healthy men. Circulation. 2000;101:1767–1772.
6. Van Dooren FEP, Nefs G, Schram MT, Verhey FRJ, Denollet J, Pouwer F. Depression and Risk of Mortality in People with Diabetes Mellitus: A Systematic Review and Meta-Analysis. Berthold HK, ed. PLoS ONE. 2013;8(3): e57058.

7. Joseph NT, Kamarck TW, Muldoon MF, Manuck SB. Daily Marital Interaction Quality and Carotid Artery Intima Medial Thickness in Healthy Middle Aged Adults. Psychosomatic medicine. 2014;76(5):347-354.

8. van den Oord SCH, Sijbrands EJG, ten Kate GL, van Klaveren D, van Domburg RT, van der Steen AFW, et al. Carotid intima-media thickness for cardiovascular risk assessment: systematic review and meta-analysis. Atherosclerosis. 2013;228:1–11.

9. Hershfield HE, Scheibe S, Sims TL, Carstensen LL. When Feeling Bad Can Be Good: Mixed Emotions Benefit Physical Health Across Adulthood. Soc Psychol Personal Sci. 2013;4(1):54–61.

57. NICOTINE: SMOKELESS TOBACCO

Introduction

It is estimated that almost 1.3 billion people smoke or use other tobacco products, including smokeless tobacco.[1] There are about 8.1 million smokeless tobacco product users in the USA.[2] Smokeless tobacco products are available in many forms, but the most commonly used are snuff (moist and dry) and chewing tobacco. They are usually held in the mouth, cheek, or lip or chewed to allow absorption of nicotine across the buccal mucosa.[3] Nicotine is the principal alkaloid found in these smokeless tobacco products, and is similar in amount in oral snuff and cigarette tobacco. Nicotine content is somewhat lower in chewing tobacco.[4]

Scientific Evidence

- Two meta-analysis evaluating the risk of cardiovascular diseases in people using smokeless tobacco found a slightly increased risk of 0.6% for heart disease and 13% for fatal heart attack.[5,6]

- Data from studies also indicates that use of smokeless tobacco increases the risk of stroke. The meta-analysis revealed an increase in this risk by 40%-42%.[5,6]

- Swedish studies reveal that, heavy use of moist snuff increases the risk of developing metabolic syndrome and type 2 diabetes.[7,8]

- Smokeless tobacco users get as much nicotine per day as do regular smokers, with the nicotine being absorbed slower in the former. Nicotine has many deleterious cardiovascular effects, including constriction of the coronary arteries and impairment of the vascular endothelial function.

- Smokeless tobacco users have a lower risk of cardiovascular morbidity and mortality and have longer life spans when compared to cigarette smokers.[9] However, smokeless tobacco is still a source of harmful carcinogens and may adversely effect the reproductive organs.[10]

Conclusion

Use of smokeless tobacco may generate reduced cardiovascular risks, when compared to smoking cigarettes. It should not be used as an alternative to cigarette smoking or as a smoking cessation product without a green signal from your health care provider. It is addictive and quitting smokeless tobacco use may be as difficult as cigarette smoking cessation.

Lifestyle Implications

Smokeless tobacco is addictive and not without cardiovascular risk. It should be avoided.

References

1. World Health Organization. Tobacco: Deadly in Any Form or Disguise. Geneva, Switzerland: World Health Organization; 2006. Accessed February 4, 2010.
2. Results from the 2008 National Survey on Drug Use and Health: National Findings. Rockville, MD: SAMHSA, Office of Applied Studies; 2009. NSDUH Series H-36, HHS Publication No. SMA 09-4434.
3. National Cancer Institute, Centers for Disease Control and Prevention, and Stockholm Centre of Public Health. Smokeless Tobacco Fact Sheets. 3rd International Conference on Smokeless Tobacco, September 20–25, 2002. Available at: http://www.cancercontrol.cancer.gov/tcrb/stfact_sheet_combined10-23-02.pdf.
4. Djordjevic MV, Doran KA. Nicotine content and delivery across tobacco products. Handb Exp Pharmacol. 2009;192:61–82.
5. Lee PN. Circulatory disease and smokeless tobacco in western populations: a review of the evidence. Int J Epidemiol. 2007;36:789–804.
6. Boffetta P, Straif K. Use of smokeless tobacco and risk of myocardial infarction and stroke: systematic review with meta-analysis. BMJ. 2009; 339:b3060.
7. Norberg M, Stenlund H, Lindahl B, Boman K, Weinehall L. Contribution of Swedish moist snuff to the metabolic syndrome: a wolf in sheep's clothing? Scand J Public Health. 2006;34:576–583.
8. Persson PG, Carlsson S, Svanstrom L, Ostenson CG, Ependic S, Grill V. Cigarette smoking, orka mosit snuff use and glucose intolerance. J Intern Med. 2000;248:103–110.
9. Teo KK, Ounpuu S, Hawken S, Pandey MR, Valentin V, Hunt D, Diaz R, Rashed W, Freeman R, Jiang L, Zhang X, Yusuf S, INTERHEART Study Investigators. Tobacco use and risk of myocardial infarction in 52 countries in the INTERHEART study: a case-control study. Lancet. 2006;368:647–658.
10. Hatsukami DK, Severson HH. Oral spit tobacco: addiction, prevention and treatment. Nicotine Tob Res.1999;1:21–44.

58. NOISE POLLUTION

Introduction

Excessive noise exposure at work due to machines or listerning to loud music during is known to damage hearing. However, the role of noise pollution or noise disturbance on having detrimental effects on other aspects of human health are not well known. Transportation - road traffic, railways and aircraft, are common causes of outdoor noise. Air pollution is known to accelerate the development of atherosclerosis and increase cardiopulmonary mortality, but is often associated with elevated noise pollution.[1] Sound pollution, by itself, also increases cardiovascular diseases and decreases the quality of life.

Scientific Evidence

- Several epidemiological studies have implicated traffic noise in the increased incidence of coronary artery disease, hypertension and stroke.[2] A recent study showed that men, exposed to sound levels of more than 70 dB(A) during the day, had a 1.3-fold increase in risk for myocardial infarction.[3]

- Chronic exposure to excessive noise at workplace has also been noted to increase cardiovascular mortality. In a study done on a group of 27,464 blue-collar workers who worked for at least one year, at 14 lumber mills in British Columbia, and followed between 1950 and 1995, researchers found that the group with the highest exposure to noise, ended up having 50% higher heart attack related deaths.[4]

- The rate of high blood pressure and heart failure also go up with increasing noise exposure. This association was confirmed in a study involving 104,145 cases of heart failure and/or hypertensive heart disease patients, followed during the years 2006-10 and compared with 654,172 control subjects in Germany.[5] There is also an increase in the rates of stroke with exposure to noise from different sources.[6]

- High noise exposure may increase the risk of developing type 2 diabetes – a major risk factor for cardiovascular diseases.[7]

- Noise results in annoyance, depression and sleep disturbance, which also contribute to an increase in cardiovascular disease.[8]

- In a study of aircraft noise related stress in mice, the increased blood pressure and vascular dysfunction caused by noise appeared to be associated with a raised level of oxidative stress.[9]
- A study of 1,244 participants older than 18 years of age and exposed to aircraft noise had their saliva cortisol measured. Data from this study revealed that excessive noise modifies the cortisol circadian rhythm and this is detrimental for the cardiovascular health. There are also harmful effects noted on the cardiovascular system mediated via the inflammatory and immune processes.[10]

Conclusion

Noise is pervasive in our environment. However, excessive noise has detrimental effects not only on the hearing but also on other bodily systems. Traffic noise (road, railway or aircraft), neighborhood noise, and other noise pollution, appear to increase the incidence of high blood pressure, stroke and coronary heart disease. Noise pollution may be as dangerous as air pollution when it comes to human cardiovascular health.

Lifestyle Implications

Long term exposure to disturbing high environmental noise, especially that from road traffic, railways or aircraft, is dangerous for your cardiovascular system.

References

1. Barbara Hoffmann, Susanne Moebus, Andreas Stang, et al. Residence close to high traffic and prevalence of coronary heart disease. Eur Heart J (2006) 27 (22): 2696-2702.
2. Héritier H, Vienneau D, Foraster M, et al. Transportation noise exposure and cardiovascular mortality: a nationwide cohort study from Switzerland. Eur J Epidemiol. 2017 Mar 9.
3. Babisch WF, Beule B, Schust M, Kersten N, Ising H. Traffic noise and risk of myocardial infarction, Epidemiology, 2005, vol. 16 (pg. 33-40)
4. Davies HW, Teschke K, Kennedy SM, et al. Occupational exposure to noise and mortality from acute myocardial infarction, Epidemiology, 2005, vol. 16: 25-32.
5. Seidler A, Wagner M, Schubert M, et al. Aircraft, road and railway traffic noise as risk factors for heart failure and hypertensive heart disease-A case-control study based on secondary data. Int J Hyg Environ Health. 2016 Nov;219(8):749-758.

6. Vandasova Z, Vencálek O, Puklová V. Specific and combined subjective responses to noise and their association with cardiovascular diseases. Noise Health. 2016 Nov-Dec;18(85):338-346.

7. Angel Mario Dzhambov. Longterm noise exposure and the risk for type 2 diabetes: A metaanalysis. Noise Health. 2015 JanFeb; 17(74): 23–33.

8. Babisch W. Transportation noise and cardiovascular risk: Updated review and synthesis of epidemiological studies indicate that the evidence has increased. Noise Health. 2006;8:1–29.

9. Münzel T, Daiber A, Steven S, et al. Effects of noise on vascular function, oxidative stress, and inflammation: mechanistic insight from studies in mice. Eur Heart J. 2017 Feb 17.

10. Alberto Recio, Cristina Linares, José Ramón Banegas, Julio Díaz. Road traffic noise effects on cardiovascular, respiratory, and metabolic health: An integrative model of biological mechanisms. Environmental Research 146 (2016) 359–370.

59. NUTS

Introduction

Nuts (especially tree nuts and peanuts) are nutrient dense foods, rich in unsaturated fatty acids and other beneficial bioactive compounds including high-quality vegetable protein, fiber, minerals, tocopherols, phytosterols, and phenolic compounds. They are a good source of nutrition and confer many positive health outcomes. Several epidemiological studies have shown that regular tree nut consumption is associated with a reduction in all-cause mortality and ischemic heart disease.[1] Several large epidemiological studies have found a protective action of frequent nut consumption on coronary heart disease.

Scientific Evidence

- In the 31,208 participants enrolled in the Adventist Health Study, subjects in the highest nut intake group had an approximate 35% lesser risk of coronary heart disease when compared to those in the lowest intake group.[2]
- Regular nut consumption was associated with a lower risk of sudden cardiac death and other coronary heart disease end points among 21,454 male participants enrolled in the US Physicians' Health Study and followed for an average of 17 years.[3]
- Nut consumption was associated with a decreased body mass index, waist circumference and systolic blood pressure (all cardiovascular risk factors) when compared with non-consumers.[4]
- Nut consumption results in a decreased prevalence of type 2 diabetes – another cardiovascular risk factor.[5] Patients with diabetes also reduce their risk and incidence of cardiovascular events with regular nut consumption. This was demonstrated in a study of 6,309 women with type 2 diabetes, with 54,656 person-years of follow-up, during which time there were 452 coronary heart disease events and 182 incident strokes. After analysis of the data, researchers concluded that frequent nut and peanut butter consumption was inversely associated with the total cardiovascular disease risk.[6]
- Tree nuts including peanuts, are nutrient dense foods with complex matrices rich in protein, fiber, unsaturated fatty acids, bioactive

polyphenolic compounds, minerals and several other micronutrients. These bioactive constituents confer significant cardio-protective effects. Nut intake is associated with positive changes in several cardiac biomarkers, such as a reduction in total and low-density lipoprotein cholesterol levels, improved low-density lipoprotein cholesterol/high-density lipoprotein cholesterol ratio, decreased low-density lipoprotein cholesterol oxidizability, reduced inflammation and improved endothelial function.

Conclusion

Epidemiological and dietary intervention data provides compelling evidence that consuming an ounce or more of nuts a week is associated with cardiovascular protection. The following equal one ounce: 24 almonds, 14 English walnut halves, 15 pecan halves, 12 macadamia nuts, 18 medium cashews, 12 hazelnuts or filberts, 35 peanuts or 8 medium Brazil nuts. A one-ounce serving of nuts contains between 160 and 200 calories.

Lifestyle Implications

Eating an ounce or more of tree nuts a week is cardioprotective.

References

1. Sabate J. Nut consumption, vegetarian diets, ischemic heart disease risk, and all-cause mortality: evidence from epidemiologic studies. Am J Clin Nutr. 1999, 70, S500-3
2. Fraser GE, Sabate J, Beeson WL, Strahan TM. A possible protective effect of nut consumption on risk of coronary heart disease. The Adventist Health Study. Arch Intern Med. 1992, 152, 1416-24.
3. Albert CM, Gaziano M, Willett WC, Manson JE. Nut consumption and decreased risk of sudden cardiac death in the Physicians' Health Study. Arch. Intern. Med. 2002, 162, 1382.
4. O'Neil CE, Keast DR, Nicklas TA, Fulgoni VL 3rd. Nut consumption is associated with decreased health risk factors for cardiovascular disease and metabolic syndrome in U.S. adults: NHANES 1999-2004. J Am Coll Nutr. 2011, 30(6), 502-10.
5. Jiang R, Manson JE, Stampfer MJ, Liu S, Willett WC, Hu FB. Nut and peanut butter consumption and risk of type 2 diabetes in women. JAMA. 2002, 288(20), 2554-603.3.2.
6. Li TY, Brennan AM, Wedick NM, Mantzoros C, Rifai N, Hu FB. Regular Consumption of Nuts Is Associated with a Lower Risk of Cardiovascular Disease in Women with Type 2 Diabetes. The Journal of Nutrition. 2009;139(7):1333-1338.

60. OLIVE OIL

Introduction

Olive oil is obtained from olives - fruits of the tree, *Olea europaea.* These trees are common in the Mediterranean basin, where they have been grown since the 8th millennium BC. The world's largest producers of olive oil are Spain, Italy and Greece. Besides its use in cooking and as a salad dressing, olive oil is used for many other non-culinary purposes, including in the manufacture of cosmetics, pharmaceuticals, and soaps. However, its popularity soared after it was recognized from epidemiological studies, that the incidence of coronary heart disease was low in countries that routinely use olive oil in their diets. Olive oil is the main fat in the Mediterranean diet and consists mainly of oleic acid (up to 83%), linoleic acid (up to 21%) and palmitic acid (up to 20%). Consumption of olive oil appears to be one of the major reasons behind the Mediterranean cardiovascular paradox – a low cardiovascular mortality despite a high prevalence of classical cardiovascular risk factors.

Scientific Evidence

- In a study of 1,128 men and 1,154 women older than 18 years, consumption of the Mediterranean diet was associated with a 26% lower risk of having high blood pressure.[1]
- the ATTICA study of 1,926 adult men and women, consumption of the Mediterranean diet was associated with a 35% reduction of coronary heart disease risk in subjects with the metabolic syndrome.[2]
- In the CARDIO2000 study, the Mediterranean diet was associated with an adjusted 23% rate reduction in the risk of developing a first event of acute coronary syndrome.[3]
- Compared to patients on AHA Set I diet, those following Mediterranean diet had a 50%-70% lower risk of recurrent heart disease.[4]
- The Healthy Ageing Study showed that a Mediterranean diet was associated with 23% lower risk of death.[5]
- Olive oil is rich in the beneficial mono-unsaturated fatty acids. These and other beneficial bioactive compounds in olive oil lead to

significant improvements in the levels of harmful biomarkers of cardiovascular disease in humans. Benefits include a decrease in low-density lipoprotein cholesterol levels, a better postprandial glucose profile, a reduced insulin and triglyceride response, decreased thrombosis, diminished inflammation, decreased oxidative stress and an improvement in endothelial function. These actions result in reduced atherosclerosis. These findings are well described in a review on olive oil and the cardiovascular system by Mar'ıa-Isabel Covas in 2007.[6]

Conclusion

Evidence based data provides compelling evidence that replacing other cooking oils or saturated fats with olive oil results in significant cardiovascular protection. Olive oil is readily available and tastes good. The recommended dose of 2 tablespoons (23 grams) of olive oil daily has been shown to reduce the risk of coronary heart disease.

Lifestyle Implications

Ensure an intake of 2 tablespoons (23 grams) of olive oil daily.

References

1. Panagiotakos, Demosthenes B; Pitsavos, et al. Status and management of hypertension in Greece: role of the adoption of a Mediterranean diet: the Attica study. Journal of Hypertension: August 2003 - Volume 21 - Issue 8 - pp 1483-1489.
2. Pitsavos C, Panagiotakos DB, Chrysohoou C, Papaioannou I, Papadimitriou L, Tousoulis D, Stefanadis C, Toutouzas P. The adoption of Mediterranean diet attenuates the development of acute coronary syndromes in people with the metabolic syndrome. Nutr J. 2003, 2, 1.
3. Panagiotakos DB, Chrysohoou C, Pitsavos C, Tzioumis K, Papaioannou I, Stefanadis C, Toutouzas P. The association of Mediterranean diet with lower risk of acute coronary syndromes, in hypertensive subjects. Int J Cardiol. 2002, 82, 141–7.
4. de Lorgeril M, Salen P, Martin JL, Monjaud I, Delaye J, Mamelle N. Mediterranean diet, traditional risk factors and the rate of cardiovascular complications after myocardial infarction. Final report of the Lyon Diet Heart Study. Circulation, 1999, 99, 779–85.
5. Knoops KT, de Groot LC, Kromhout D, Perrin AE, MoreirasVarela O, Menotti A, van Staveren WA. Mediterranean Diet, Lifestyle Factors, and 10-Year Mortality in Elderly European Men and Women: The HALE Project. JAMA. 2004, 292(12), 1433-1439.

6. Mar´ıa-Isabel Covas. Olive oil and the cardiovascular system.
    Pharmacological Research 2007, 55, 175–186.

61. PETS

Introduction

The American Veterinary Medical Association estimates that in 2012, 36.5 % of the US households owned dogs, 30.4 % owned cats, 3.1 % owned birds, and 1.5 % owned horses. Overall there were almost 70 million dogs and 74 million cats living with Americans.[1] Pets may also help increase physical activity and thereby reduce cardiovascular risk. Other protective factors, particularly a reduction in negative emotions, also play a role.

Scientific Evidence

- Pet owners have lower cardiovascular risk factors.[2]
- In a study of 92 survivors of myocardial infarction or angina pectoris, having a pet increased the one-year survival to 94 % as compared to 72 % among those who were not pet owners.[3] Pets not only helped increase physical activity but also helped reduce depression in their owners. In a subsequent study of 460 participants following a myocardial infarction and followed for a median of 2.8 years, Friedmann and associates also found that pet ownership was associated with lower mortality.[4]
- In a large study spanning 20 years on the risk of death due to cardiovascular events such as myocardial infarction, combined cardiovascular disease stroke and that from all-causes, and its relationship with pet ownership, researches concluded that pet ownership was cardioprotective. Of the 4,435 participants in this study, 2,435 (55 %) were current or past owners of cats. Past cat ownership was associated with a significant 37 % lower risk of fatal myocardial infarction They postulate that the protective effect was related to a relaxing effect on autonomic reactivity. It is also possible that the personalities of cat owners may be protective toward cardiovascular disease.[5]
- Dog ownership is also cardiovascular protective. An examination of 916 people over the age of 18 years compared cardiovascular risk factors in three separate groups: owners who walked their dogs, owner who did not walk them, or non-dog owners. This cross-sectional study composed largely of educated white women showed that those who did not own dogs had greater odds of self-

reported diabetes, hypertension, and hypercholesterolemia when compared to those who regularly walked their dogs.[6]

- Pet owners are more active, and this helps in reducing their blood pressure, plasma cholesterol and triglycerides. They demonstrate improved survival following a myocardial infarction when compared to non-pet owners.[7]

- Psychological stress has a negative impact on the heart and accounts for more than 30 % of the attributable risk for acute myocardial infarction.[8] (Das et al, 2006). Pet owners have less stress, depression, hostility, anxiety, and isolation. These negative emotions lead to chronic autonomic imbalance, abdominal obesity, increased cortisol, and other physiological effects, leading to adverse cardiovascular results. Pets help reduce these risk factors.

Conclusion

Pet ownership is a common way to find companionship, increase activity and abolish negative emotions. There are significant cardiovascular benefits also. Both cats and dogs as pets show improved cardiovascular profiles in their owners. Dog owners may have a slight advantage, because they end up being more active. Overall, pets improve heath and the quality of life.

Lifestyle Implications

Own a pet. Both the pet and you will be happier. And you will have less cardiovascular disease!

References

1. U.S. Pet Ownership & Demographics Sourcebook. 2012 https://www.avma.org/kb/resources/statistics/pages/market-research-statistics-us-pet-ownership-demographics-sourcebook.aspx.
2. Anderson WP, Reid CM, Jennings GL. Pet owners have lower levels of accepted risk factors for cardiovascular disease. Med J Aust. 1992 Sep 7;157(5):298-301.
3. Friedmann E, Katcher AH, Lynch JL, Thomas SA. Animal companions and one-year survival of patients after discharge from a coronary care unit. Public Health Rep. 1980;95(4):307–12.
4. Friedmann E, Thomas SA, H S, for the HAT Investigators Pets, depression and long-term survival in community living patients following myocardial infarction. Anthrozoös. 2011;24(3):273–85.
5. Qureshi AI, Memon MA, Vazquez G, Suri MFK. Cat ownership and risk of fatal cardiovascular diseases. Results from the second national health

and nutrition examination study mortality follow-up study. J Vasc Interv Neurol. 2009;2(1):132–5.

6. Lentino C, Visek AJ, McDonnell K, DiPietro L. Dog walking is associated with a favorable risk profile independent of a moderate to high volume of physical activity. J Phys Act Health. 2012;9:414–20.

7. Arhant-Sudhir K, Arhant-Sudhir R, Sudhir K. Pet ownership and cardiovascular risk reduction: supporting evidence, conflicting data and underlying mechanisms. Clin Exp Pharmacol Physiol. 2011 Nov;38(11):734-8.

8. Das S, O'Keefe JH. Behavioral cardiology: recognizing and addressing the profound impact of psychosocial stress on cardiovascular health. Curr Atheroscler Rep. 2006;8:111–8.

62. POLLUTION: AIR

Introduction

Air pollution is detrimental for our health,[1] and is a major preventable environmental risk. It is estimated that in 2008, nearly 1.3 million deaths in the world were related to ambient air pollution and two million to household air pollution. In 2012, the World Health Organization (WHO) recorded an increase to nearly seven million deaths from combined ambient and household air pollution. Despite several governmental interventions. these numbers continue to climb. Besides ambient air pollution, indoor air pollution also poses a major health risk to over 3 billion people who use solid fuels such as wood, charcoal, coal, dung and crop wastes to cook and heat their homes. WHO estimates that 4.3 million people die each year from exposure to household air pollution. Air pollution has a major negative impact on the health, especially the pulmonary and digestive system. It also affects the cardiovascular system, and is responsible for a significant number of cardiovascular events and deaths.[2] Particulate matter in the environment is primarily divided into three categories according to their aerodynamic diameter: coarse: $PM_{10} - PM_{2.5}$; fine: $PM_{2.5}$ to PM_1 and ultrafine: $<PM_1$. Most studies show that $PM_{2.5}$ particles play a major role in cardiovascular morbidity and mortality.[3]

Scientific Evidence

- A considerable epidemiological and clinical data substantiates that both short term and long-term exposure to air pollution is detrimental to human health. Increased particulate matter pollution results in exacerbations in the symptoms of cardiovascular diseases, and increases in emergency room visits and hospital admissions.[4]

- There is an increase in the incidence of ischemic strokes.[5] Stroke related hospitalizations and deaths also increase as the air pollution gets worse.[6]

- There is worsening of heart failure in patients, resulting in an increase in heart failure hospitalizations and an increase in heart failure mortality.[7]

- Patients dying of sudden cardiac death appear to do so more when ambient air pollution is high.[8]

- There is an increase in deaths related to coronary artery disease, with an increase in air pollution.[9] Overall, increasing air pollution results in increased cardiovascular morbidity and mortality.[10] The life expectancy is reduced.

- Particulate air pollutants affect the cardiovascular system in many ways. They cause endothelial dysfunction and vasoconstriction, increase blood pressure and heart rate, increase prothrombotic and coagulant activity, increase systemic inflammation, and oxidative stress responses. They decrease heart rate variability, increase autonomic imbalance, induce arrhythmias, raise insulin resistance, and lead to the progression of atherosclerosis.

Conclusions

Particulate air pollution, is strongly associated with a host of medical ailments, including an increase in cardiovascular morbidity and mortality. A reduction in the particulate matter in the ambient and household air decreases disease exacerbations, emergency room visits, hospitalizations and premature death.

Lifestyle Implications

Breathe clean air, both indoors and outdoors. It will keep your cardiovascular system clean.

References

1. Lai H-K, Tsang H, Wong C-M. Meta-analysis of adverse health effects due to air pollution in Chinese populations. BMC Public Health. 2013; 13:360.
2. www.who.int
3. Pope CA 3rd, Dockery DW. Health effects of fine particulate air pollution: lines that connect. J Air Waste Manag Assoc. 2006; 56: 709–742.
4. Ito K, Mathes R, Ross Z, Nádas A, Thurston G, Matte T. Fine Particulate Matter Constituents Associated with Cardiovascular Hospitalizations and Mortality in New York City. Environmental Health Perspectives. 2011;119(4):467-473.
5. Ljungman PL, Mittleman MA. Ambient Air Pollution and Stroke. Stroke; a journal of cerebral circulation. 2014;45(12):3734-3741.
6. Shah ASV, Lee KK, McAllister DA, et al. Short term exposure to air pollution and stroke: systematic review and meta-analysis. The BMJ. 2015;350:h1295.

7. Shah AS, Langrish JP, Nair H, et al. Global association of air pollution and heart failure: a systematic review and meta-analysis. Lancet. 2013;382(9897):1039-1048.

8. Wichmann J, Folke F, Torp-Pedersen C, et al. Out-of-Hospital Cardiac Arrests and Outdoor Air Pollution Exposure in Copenhagen, Denmark. ten Cate H, ed. PLoS ONE. 2013;8(1): e53684.

9. Hoek G, Krishnan RM, Beelen R, et al. Long-term air pollution exposure and cardio- respiratory mortality: a review. Environmental Health. 2013;12:43.

10. Guo Y, Li S, Tawatsupa B, Punnasiri K, Jaakkola JJK, Williams G. The association between air pollution and mortality in Thailand. Scientific Reports. 2014;4:5509.

63. POTASSIUM

Introduction

Potassium, symbol K (from Neo-Latin kalium) is necessary for the proper functioning of all living cells. It was identified as a shortfall nutrient by the Dietary Guidelines for Americans 2010 Advisory Committee.[1] Potassium is protective for age-related bone loss and helps in the reduction of kidney stones. Conclusive evidence also exists for the beneficial association between adequate potassium intake and blood pressure reduction in adults. Hypertension is a major risk factor for the development of stroke and coronary heart disease.

Scientific Evidence

- In a study involving a total of 586 participants, oral potassium supplements significantly lowered systolic blood pressure (mean reduction 5.9 mmHg) and diastolic blood pressure (mean reduction 3.4 mmHg).[2]

- In another meta-analysis of 33 randomized, controlled trials involving 2,609 participants with normal blood pressure, potassium supplementation was associated with a significant mean reduction of systolic blood pressure by 3.11 mm Hg and diastolic blood pressure by 1.97 mm Hg.[3] These blood pressure lowering effects were greater in blacks than whites and in hypertensives than normotensives.

- It is estimated that increasing potassium intake would decrease the incidence of hypertension in Americans by 17% and would increase life expectancy by 5.1 years.[4]

- A dietary intake of >3500 mg/d is recommended for the primary prevention of hypertension.[5]

- In a review of eleven studies with 247,510 male and female participants (followed for 5 to 19 years), researchers recorded 7,066 strokes, 3,058 coronary heart disease events, and 2,497 total cardiovascular disease events. A meta-analysis revealed a reduction in the risk of stroke by 21% for every 1.64-g/day increase in potassium intake. Beneficial trends towards a lower risk of cardiovascular disease were also noted.[6]

- A potassium rich diet may also help reduce the risk of developing diabetes mellitus.[7]
- Potassium exerts its antihypertensive effects via several mechanisms, including a reduction of intravascular volume and an increased endothelium-dependent vasodilation. Other complex mechanisms also come into play.

Conclusions

Potassium is an important element that is found in fruits and vegetables. Potatoes are a good source. However, potassium is not typically found in fortified foods and is not commonly consumed as a dietary supplement. Current recommendations are of 4,700 mg/day but clinical trials on blood pressure suggest 3,600–3,800 mg/day may be cardioprotective. Oral potassium supplements come with the risk of high potassium blood levels, which can be dangerous.[8] It is therefore, best to increase potassium intake via foods rather than supplements.[1] Besides potatoes, other good sources of potassium include milk, coffee, chicken, beef, and orange and grapefruit juice.

Lifestyle Implications

Adequate potassium intake, especially from an increased consumption of potassium rich foods, is cardioprotective.

References

1. Dietary Guidelines Advisory Committee Report of the Dietary Guidelines Advisory Committee on the Dietary Guidelines for Americans, 2010. Washington, DC: U.S. Department of Agriculture, Agricultural Research Service, 2011.
2. Cappuccio FP, MacGregor GA. Does potassium supplementation lower blood pressure? A meta-analysis of published trials. J Hypertens. 1991;9:465–73.
3. Whelton PK, He J, Cutler JA, Brancati FL, Appel LJ, Follman D, Klag MJ. Effect of oral potassium on blood pressure. JAMA. 1997;277:1624–32.
4. Roger VL, Go AS, Lloyd-Jones DM, Benjamin EJ, Berry JD, Borden WB, Bravata DM, Dai S, Ford ES, Fox CS, et al., on behalf of the American Heart Association Statistics Committee and Stroke Statistics Subcommittee Heart disease and stroke statistics – 2012 update: a report from the American Heart Association. Circulation. 2012;125: e2–220.

5. Chobanian AV, Bakris GL, Black HR, Cushman WC, Green LA, Izzo JL, Jr, Jones DW, Materson BJ, Oparil S, Wright JT, Jr, et al. the National High Blood Pressure Education Program Coordinating Committee. The Seventh Report of the Joint National Committee on Prevention, Detection, Evaluation, and Treatment of High Blood Pressure: The JNC 7 report. JAMA. 2003;289:2560–72.

6. D'Elia L, Barba G, Cappuccio FP, Strazzullo P. Potassium intake, stroke, and cardiovascular disease. A meta-analysis of prospective studies. J Am Coll Cardiol. 2011;57:1210–9.

7. Chatterjee R, Colangelo LA, Yeh HC, et al. Potassium intake and risk of incident type 2 diabetes mellitus: the Coronary Artery Risk Development in Young Adults (CARDIA) Study. Diabetologia. 2012;55(5):1295-1303.

8. Wang W, Soltero L, Zhang D, Huang XR, Lan HY, Adrogue HJ. Renal inflammation is modulated by potassium in chronic kidney disease: possible role of Smad 7. Am J Physiol Renal Physiol. 2007; 293:F1123–30.

64. PREDIABETES

Introduction

It is estimated that more than 84 million people in the United States have prediabetes - and 9 out of 10 of them do not know that they have it. Recent studies suggest that 1 out of 3 people over the age of 18, and almost half of the people over age 65, have prediabetes. Without lifestyle changes to improve their health, 15%-30% of people with prediabetes will develop type 2 diabetes within 5 years. Prediabetes is usually diagnosed by blood tests which measure fasting blood sugar and glycated hemoglobin (HbA1c). Normal fasting blood sugar should be less than 100 mg/dl. Prediabetes is diagnosed if the blood sugar level is between 100 to 125 mg/dL and diabetes is diagnosed if the blood sugar level is 126 mg/dl or higher. A normal HbA1c is below 5.7 percent. A level between 5.7 and 6.4 percent indicates prediabetes, while a level of 6.5 percent or higher on two separate tests indicates diabetes mellitus. Individuals with prediabetes exhibit an elevated risk of damage to the micro-vasculature and macro-vasculature, resembling the long-term complications of diabetes. Type 2 diabetes is strongly linked with a higher cardiovascular morbidity,[1] and mortality,[2] and emerging data indicates that people with prediabetes share this increased risk.

Scientific Evidence

- Patients with prediabetes have a higher presence of known cardiovascular risk factors, specifically abdominal obesity, hypertension and low high-density lipoprotein cholesterol levels.[3]
- In a study of sixty-seven patients undergoing angioscopic visualization of coronary arteries, researchers found higher coronary atherosclerosis and plaque vulnerability in prediabetic than in nondiabetic patients. These changes were comparable between prediabetic and diabetic patients.[4]
- In a review of 18 studies, researchers found that prediabetes increases the risk of cardiovascular events by 10%-20%. When comparing women and men, for any given prediabetic category, women had a greater relative risk of cardiovascular disease than

men.[6] This increased risk included increased cardiovascular and all-cause mortality.[7]

- Prediabetes patients have an increased risk of cerebrovascular diseases, such as transient ischemic attack, stroke, and recurrent stroke. In one study, almost 50% of the nondiabetic patients with a recent transient ischemic attack or stroke had prediabetes. This is more than that seen in the general population.[8]

- Progression to diabetes mellitus may be signaled by the development of increased thirst, frequent urination, fatigue and blurred vision.

Conclusion

The risk factors for prediabetes include being overweight, a large waist size (>40 in for men and >35 in for women), inactivity, increasing age, family history of diabetes or prediabetes, being of African-Americas, Hispanic, American Indian, Asian-American and Pacific Islander race, having suffered from gestational diabetes, having polycystic ovary syndrome and several sleep disorders including obstructive sleep apnea. Prediabetes is also higher in people with high blood pressure, low high-density lipoprotein cholesterol levels and high triglyceride levels. Lifestyle interventions such as eating proper diet, maintaining optimal body weight and regular exercise, help reduce the progression to overt type 2 diabetes by 58 percent over 2.8 years.

Lifestyle Implications

Prediabetes is associated with increased cardiovascular events. Maintain an optimal body weight, eat a proper diet and participate in a regular exercise program.

References

1. DeFronzo RA, Abdul-Ghani M. Assessment and treatment of cardiovascular risk in prediabetes: impaired glucose tolerance and impaired fasting glucose. Am J Cardiol. 2011;108:3B–24B.
2. Barr EL, Zimmet PZ, Welborn TA, et al. Risk of cardiovascular and all-cause mortality in individuals with diabetes mellitus, impaired fasting glucose, and impaired glucose tolerance: the Australian Diabetes, Obesity, and Lifestyle Study (AusDiab) Circulation. 2007;116:151–157.
3. Díaz-Redondo A, Giráldez-García C, Carrillo L, et al. Modifiable risk factors associated with prediabetes in men and women: a cross-sectional analysis of the cohort study in primary health care on the evolution of

patients with prediabetes (PREDAPS-Study). BMC Family Practice. 2015;16:5.

4. Kurihara O, Takano M, Yamamoto M, et al. Impact of Prediabetic Status on Coronary Atherosclerosis: A multivessel angioscopic study. Diabetes Care. 2013;36(3):729-733.

5. Ford ES, Zhao G, Li C. Pre-diabetes and the risk for cardiovascular disease: a systematic review of the evidence. J Am Coll Cardiol. 2010 3-30;55(13):1310-7.

6. Yamini S. Levitzky, Michael J. Pencina, et al. Impact of Impaired Fasting Glucose on Cardiovascular Disease. JACC, 2008. Volume 51, Issue 3, Pages 264-270.

7. Huang Y, Cai X, Mai W, Li M, Hu Y. Association between prediabetes and risk of cardiovascular disease and all cause mortality: systematic review and meta-analysis. The BMJ. 2016;355: i5953.

8. Fonville S, Zandbergen AA, Koudstaal PJ, den Hertog HM. Prediabetes in patients with stroke or transient ischemic attack: prevalence, risk and clinical management. Cerebrovasc Dis. 2014;37(6):393–400.

9. Katula JA, Vitolins MZ, Morgan TM, The Healthy Living Partnerships to Prevent Diabetes Study: 2-year outcomes of a randomized controlled trial. Am J Prev Med. 2013;44(Suppl 4): S324-S332.

65. PROTEIN

Introduction

Epidemiologic studies show an inverse relationship between increased protein intake, especially from plant sources, and a lower risk of hypertension and coronary heart disease. Higher protein intake from red meat, specifically beef and pork, and from processed meat, has the reverse effect.

Scientific Evidence

- It has been noted that high-protein diets enhance weight loss.[1] High protein intake increases diet-induced thermogenesis and satiety and results in decreased hunger.[2]
- Higher consumption of dietary protein is inversely associated with blood pressure in several studies and animal experiments. The benefits are more prominent with the intake of plant protein.[3]
- Increasing protein intake and decreasing carbohydrate intake helps improve the cholesterol profile. In one study, patients with high cholesterol levels were assigned either to a high-protein (23% energy) and low-carbohydrate (53% energy) diet or low-protein (11% energy) and high-carbohydrate (65% energy) diet for 4–5 weeks. Protein sources included turkey, cottage cheese, beef, fish, and ham. Researchers noticed a significantly reduced low density lipoprotein cholesterol (by 6.4%) and triacylglycerol (by 23%) levels and increased high-density lipoprotein cholesterol (by 12%) in the high protein group.[4]
- In the Nurses' Health Study, Hu and associates found that people consuming the most protein (highest quintile – 24% energy from protein) had a 36% lower risk of coronary heart disease when compared to those eating the least protein (lowest quintile – 15% energy from protein).[5]
- There are suggestions in the scientific literature that high protein intake may be associated with a decreased risk of stroke, especially hemorrhagic stroke.

Conclusions

Centers for Disease Control and Prevention recommends that protein
intake be between 10 percent to 35 percent of the daily calories. According
to the American Heart Associaton, consumption of an 8-ounce glass of
milk (8 grams of protein), a cup of yogurt (11 grams), a 3-ounce piece of
meat (21 grams), and a cup of dry beans (16 grams), may help reach the 56-
gram requirement for an adult man.[6]

Lifestyle Implications

*Adequate protein consumption may be cardioprotective, especially if the protein is of plant
origin. Opt for low-fat sources of proteins, such as lean meats, skim milk, legumes, low
fat yogurt etc.*

References

1. Larsen TM, Dalskov SM, van Baak M, Jebb SA, Papadaki A, Pfeiffer AF,
    Martinez JA, Handjieva-Darlenska T, Kunšová M, Pihlsgård M, et al.
    Diet, Obesity, and Genes (DIOgenes) Project. Diets with high or low
    protein content and glycemic index for weight-loss maintenance. N Engl J
    Med. 2010;363:2102–13.
2. Halton TL, Hu FB. The effects of high protein diets on thermogenesis,
    satiety and weight loss: a critical review. J Am Coll Nutr 2004;23:373–85.
3. Appel LJ. The effects of protein intake on blood pressure and
    cardiovascular disease. Curr Opin Lipidol. 2003 Feb;14(1):55-9.
4. Wolfe BM, Giovannetti PM. Short-term effects of substituting protein for
    carbohydrate in the diets of moderately hypercholesterolemic human
    subjects. Metabolism 1991;40:338–43.
5. Hu FB, Stampfer MJ, Manson JE, et al. Dietary protein and risk of
    ischemic heart disease in women. Am J Clin Nutr 1999;70:221–7.
6. http://www.heart.org/HEARTORG/Conditions/More/MyHeartandStr
    okeNews/Protein-and-Heart-
    Health_UCM_434962_Article.jsp#.WZdV3yiGPAw

66. RED/PROCESSED MEAT

Introduction

Red meat is usually referred to muscle meat such as that from beef, veal, pork, lamb, horse, deer and some types of game. Certain parts of chicken and the muscle tissue of ducks and geese are also red meat. This meat is usually made of slow twitch fibers. Red meat also has a myoglobin count higher than 65%. White meat usually refers to poultry, fish, amphibians, and reptiles, is lighter in color and is mainly made of fast twitch fibers." Processed meat" refers to meat, with added water, salts and other compounds, mainly to extend their shelf life. These include bacon, hot dogs, sausages, cold cuts and other predominantly red meats. Red and processed meat is positively associated with an increased risk of obesity, colorectal cancer, and type II diabetes mellitus. Red meat consumption increases all-cause mortality. There is also an increased risk of cardiovascular disease, especially ischemic heart disease, and cardiovascular mortality, in these people.

Scientific Evidence

- The association of red meat intake and high blood pressure has been reported in several publications. Lajous and associates reported in 2014 that in women who consumed ≥5 servings. (50 g = 1 serving) of processed red meat/week, there was a 17% higher rate of hypertension when compared to women who consumed <1 serving/week.[1]

- In a meta-analysis of two cohort studies, Pan and his group followed 37,698 men from the Health Professionals Follow-up Study (1986-2008) and 83,644 women from the Nurses' Health Study (1980-2008). In this analysis, the cardiovascular mortality was increased by 13% for a 1-serving per day increase in consumption of unprocessed red meat, and by 12% for a similar increase in the consumption of processed red meat.[2]

- Increased consumption of red meat is associated with an increase in ischemic strokes. In a meta-analysis of five prospective cohort studies, involving a total of 2,39 251 subjects and 9,593 stroke events, Chen and associates found that the relative risk for ischemic stroke were 15% higher for total meat consumption (red and processed meat combined), 9% higher for red meat consumption and 14% higher for processed meat consumption, in the high meat consumption group when compared to the low meat consumption group.[3]

- In a prospective follow-up trial on 37,035 Swedish men, there was a 28% increase in heart failure in men consuming 1.2 servings/day of processed red meat and a 43% more increase in heart failure related deaths in those consuming 0.2 servings/day.[4] They also reported that in 2,806 women with heart failure, followed for a mean of 13.2 years, women who consumed ≥ 50 g/day processed red meat compared to those who consumed < 25 g/day, there was a statistically significant 23% higher risk of heart failure.[5]

- In a meta-analysis of several cohort studies (1,674,272 individuals), Abete and group noted a 16 % higher risk of cardiovascular mortality with red meat consumption, and a 18% higher risk of cardiovascular mortality in those with the highest category of processed meat consumption.[6]

- There are many pathways by which meat consumption can increase the risk of developing cardiovascular diseases. These include higher levels of total serum cholesterol, low-density-lipoprotein cholesterol, and triglycerides in meat eaters when compared with individuals who consumed no meat. Processed meats are higher in dietary sodium and nitrates.

Conclusion

Red meat is usually referred to the muscle meat from beef, veal, pork, lamb, horse, deer and some types of game, with a myoglobin count higher than 65%. Increased consumption of red meat, particularly processed red meat, is associated with an increased risk of a wide range of serious medical illnesses, including obesity, type II diabetes, some cancers and cardiovascular diseases. It also increases cardiovascular mortality and all-cause mortality.

Lifestyle Implications

Limit your consumption of red meat, especially processed red meat. Replace it with plant based foods.

References

1. Lajous M, Bijon A, Fagherazzi G, et al. Processed and unprocessed red meat consumption and hypertension in women. Am J Clin Nutr. 2014 Sep;100(3):948-52. doi: 10.3945/ajcn.113.080598. Epub 2014 Jul 30.

2. Pan A, Sun Q, Bernstein AM, Schulze MB, Manson JE, Stampfer MJ, Willett WC, Hu FB. Red meat consumption and mortality: results from 2 prospective cohort studies. Arch Intern Med. 2012;172:555–563.

3. Chen GC, Lv DB, Pang Z et al, Red and processed meat consumption and risk of stroke: a meta-analysis of prospective cohort studies. European Journal of Clinical Nutrition (2013) 67, 91–95.

4. Kaluza J, Åkesson A, Wolk A. Processed and unprocessed red meat consumption and risk of heart failure: prospective study of men. Circ Heart Fail. 2014;7:552–557.

5. Kaluza J, Åkesson A, Wolk A. Long-term processed and unprocessed red meat consumption and risk of heart failure: A prospective cohort study of women. Int J Cardiol. 2015 Aug 15;193:42-6.

6. Abete I, Romaguera D, Vieira AR, Lopez de Munain A, Norat T. Association between total, processed, red and white meat consumption and all-cause, CVD and IHD mortality: a meta-analysis of cohort studies. Br J Nutr. 2014 Sep 14;112(5):762-75.

67. SALT (SODIUM)

Introduction

Sodium chloride is the main mineral in table salt (common salt). It is an essential nutrient for human health. High salt intake is however associated with high blood pressure – the higher the intake, the higher the risk of developing hypertension.[1] Elevated blood pressure is associated with increased risk of cardiovascular disease.[2] High dietary sodium intake is therefore associated with increased cardiovascular morbidity and mortality.[3] The 2010 dietary guidelines for Americans recommended that the sodium intake be less than 2,300 mg/day. In higher risk people who are at least 51 years old or African-Americans or have hypertension, diabetes, or chronic kidney disease, the intake should be less than 1,500 mg/day.[4] The American Heart Association 2010 guidelines recommend sodium intake to be less than 1,500 mg/day for the entire U.S. population,[5] irrespective of their risk profile.

Scientific Evidence

- High salt intake is associated with high blood pressure.[3]
- Hypertension is detrimental to the cardiovascular system. A meta-analysis was done of 61 prospective observational studies of blood pressure and mortality. This study involved one million adults (ages 40-89 years) and 12.7 million person-years at risk, and involved about 56,000 cardio-vascular deaths (12,000 from stroke, 34,000 from ischemic heart disease and 10,000 from other vascular causes).and 66,000 non-cardiovascular deaths. Researchers concluded that high blood pressure was strongly and directly related to vascular (and overall) mortality.[6]
- High blood pressure is responsible for 62% of stroke and 49% of coronary heart disease.[3]
- A meta-analysis of thirty-four trials (3,230 participants) revealed that a modest reduction in salt intake lowered blood pressure.[7] (He et al, 2013) Another meta-analysis indicated a significant (20%) reduction in cardiovascular events with a reduction of 800 to 920 mg in sodium intake over 6 to 36 months.[8]

- Sodium also plays a major role in heart failure. The average daily intake of 4 grams of sodium a day by the USA population may be harmful to adults with heart failure.[9] The Heart Failure Society of America recommends a daily consumption of 2-3 grams or less of sodium in the heart failure population, depending on the heart failure severity.[10]

Conclusion

The association between increased salt/sodium intake and hypertension/cardiovascular disease is irrefutable. It is estimated that by reducing the average sodium intake by just 400 mg per day, there may be 28,000 fewer deaths in the USA. Worldwide, a 15% (about 1.5-2.3 g/day) reduction in mean population salt intake could avert 8.5 million cardiovascular deaths. Unfortunately, in the developed countries, majority of the sodium is already in the food before it reaches the kitchen.

Lifestyle Implications

Salt restriction to about 1500 mg/day helps reduce blood pressure and is cardiovascular system protective.

References

1. Gleibermann L. Blood pressure and dietary salt in human populations. Ecol Food Nutr (1973) 2(2):143.10.1080/03670244.1973.9990329.
2. Lewington S, Clarke R, Qizilbash N, Peto R, Collins R, Prospective Studies C. Age-specific relevance of usual blood pressure to vascular mortality: a meta-analysis of individual data for one million adults in 61 prospective studies. Lancet (2002) 360(9349):1903–13.10.1016/S0140-6736(02)11911-8.
3. He FJ, MacGregor GA. Reducing population salt intake worldwide: from evidence to implementation. Prog Cardiovasc Dis (2010) 52(5):363–82.10.1016/j.pcad.2009.12.006.
4. U.S. Department of Agriculture and U.S. Department of Health and Human Services. Dietary Guidelines for Americans, 2010. 7th ed Washington, DC: U.S. Government Printing Office.
5. Lloyd-Jones DM, Hong Y, Labarthe D, Mozaffarian D, Appel LJ, Van Horn L, et al. Defining and setting national goals for cardiovascular health promotion and disease reduction. The american heart association's strategic impact goal through 2020 and beyond. Circulation (2010) 121(4):586–613.10.1161/CIRCULATIONAHA.109.192703.

6. Lewington S, Clarke R, Qizilbash N, Peto R, Collins R; Prospective Studies Collaboration. Age-specific relevance of usual blood pressure to vascular mortality: a meta-analysis of individual data for one million adults in 61 prospective studies. Lancet. 2002 Dec 14;360(9349):1903-13.

7. He Feng J, Li Jiafu, MacGregor Graham A. Effect of longer term modest salt reduction on blood pressure: Cochrane systematic review and meta-analysis of randomised trials BMJ 2013; 346 :f1325.

8. He FJ, MacGregor GA. Salt reduction lowers cardiovascular risk: meta-analysis of outcome trials. Lancet. 2011;378:380–2.

9. Bernstein AM, Willett WC. Trends in 24-h urinary sodium excretion in the United States, 1957-2003: a systematic review. The American Journal Of Clinical Nutrition. 2010;92:1172–80.

10. Heart Failure Society of America Executive summary: HFSA 2010 comprehensive heart failure practice guideline. J Card Fail. 2010;16(6):475–539.

68. SEAWEED

Introduction

Seaweed is a term used for red, green or brown marine algae. It is commonly used in food by coastal inhabitants all over the world. It is rich in complete protein, iodine and fiber. Indonesia and the Philipines are the world's largest producers of marine seaweed. Freshwater algae are toxic and not edible, and are not used as seaweed. Some marine seaweed ingredients are also used in the manufacturing of some toothpastes, cosmetics and paints. Sea weed is also used for medicinal purposes, to prevent goiter and is often seen in diet pills. Several health benefits have been attributed to seaweed intake, including cardiovascular.[1] Scientific studies have demonstrated its beneficial role in controlling cholesterol, diabetes, hypertension, and weight. The high life expectancy of the Japanese has been partly attributed to their regular intake of these marine macroalgae.

Scientific Evidence

- Hypertensive benefits were also demonstrated in human subjects. Dried Wakame, a common seaweed in Japan, eaten for a four-week period reduced both systolic and diastolic blood pressure on an average by 14 mmHg and 5 mmHg respectively.[2] It has been noted in animal models that seaweed ingredients have an innate angiotensin converting enzyme inhibitory effect similar to several commonly used blood pressure medications.
- Seaweed helps in improving the lipid profile, especially in animal studies.[3]
- Seaweeds are also rich in long-chain omega-3 polyunsaturated fatty acids - with beneficial effects on the cardiovascular system.[4]
- Seaweed is rich in minerals.[5] These include several essential minerals such as Na, K, Mg, P, I, Zn and Fe. Magnesium is also present in marine seaweed in higher amount than in terrestrial plants and animals, and is specifically cardiovascular friendly. Both k and Mg in seaweed may help in blood pressure reduction.
- Phlorotannins in seaweed are also bioactive as anti-oxidants.[6] Fucoxanthin, is another bio-active compound that also helps by its anti-inflammatory actions.[7] Marine macroalgae are rich in fiber,[8] and this has been linked to cardiovascular protection.

- Marine algae, are rich in fucoxanthin, alginates, fucoidans and phlorotannins. These help in reducing obesity. Mechanisms include, the inhibition of lipid absorption and metabolism, an increase in the satiety feeling, and inhibition of adipocyte differentiation.[9] One double-blind human trial demonstrated an average weight loss of 4.9 kilograms in obese women who took a seaweed extract containing fucoxanthin and pomegranate seed oil for 16 weeks.

Conclusion

Many studies have demonstrated the beneficial effects of seaweed on the cardiovascular system. Depending on the type of seaweed consumed, there are reductions in obesity, hypertension and abnormal lipids. Algae also help reduce obesity, another risk factor for cardiovascular disease. Given the vast oceans with extensive shallow and reef areas where seaweed can be farmed, and its functional nutritional value, seaweed is a food that will increase in worldwide consumption in the future.

Lifestyle Implications

Eating seaweed is good for cardiovascular health.

References

1. Susana M. Cardoso, Olívia R. Pereira, Ana M. L. Seca, et al. Seaweeds as Preventive Agents for Cardiovascular Diseases: From Nutrients to Functional Foods. Mar Drugs. 2015 Nov; 13(11): 6838–6865.
2. A. Jiménez-Escrig, E. Gómez-Ordóñez, P. Rupérez. Seaweed as a Source of Novel Nutraceuticals: Sulfated Polysaccharides and Peptides. Marine Medicinal Foods — Implications and Applications, Macro and Microalgae. Volume 64, 2011, Pages 325–337. Elsevier.
3. Bahmani M., Mirhoseini M., Shirzad H., et al. A Review on Promising Natural Agents Effective on Hyperlipidemia. J. Evid. Based Comp. Altern. Med. 2015;20:228–238.
4. Pereira H, Barreira L, Figueiredo F, Custódio L, Vizetto-Duarte C, Polo C, Rešek E, Aschwin E, Varela J. Polyunsaturated fatty acids of marine macroalgae: Potential for nutritional and pharmaceutical applications. Mar. Drugs. 2012;10:1920–1935.
5. Bocanegra A., Bastida S., Benedí J., Ródenas S., Sánchez-Muniz F.J. Characteristics and nutritional and cardiovascular-health properties of seaweeds. J. Med. Food. 2009;12:236–258.

6.   Costa-Mugica A., Batista-Gonzalez A.E., Mondejar D., et al. Inhibition of LDL-oxidation and antioxidant properties related to polyphenol content of hydrophilic fractions from seaweed Halimeda Incrassata (Ellis) Lamouroux. Brazilian J. Pharm. Sci. 2012;48:31–37.

7.   Lihn A.S., Pedersen S.B., Richelsen B. Adiponectin: Action, regulation and association to insulin sensitivity. Obes. Rev. 2005;6:13–21.

8.   Dawczynski C., Schubert R., Jahreis G. Amino acids, fatty acids, and dietary fibre in edible seaweed products. Food Chem. 2007;103:891–899.

9.   Chu Wan-Loy and Phang Siew-Moi. Marine Algae as a Potential Source for Anti-Obesity Agents. Mar. Drugs 2016, 14, 222.

69. SECOND HAND SMOKE

Introduction

Second hand smoke is a mixture of mainstream smoke exhaled by the smoker and side stream smoke expelled from the end of a lit cigarette. It is composed of thousands of toxic and carcinogenic compounds.[1] These compounds include nicotine and particulate matter. Second hand smoke causes premature death and disease, especially from respiratory disease and lung cancer. There also exert harmful effects in children and these include increased lower respiratory infection, asthma, acute otitis media, sudden infant death syndrome, and higher school absenteeism.[2] Significant cardiovascular changes also occur, and in one study, implementation of the smoke free laws reduced acute myocardial infarction incidence by approximately 10%. [3] According to the world health organizaton, 1.0% of the entire worldwide mortality or 603,000 deaths was attributed to second hand smoke exposure in 2004.

Scientific Evidence

- A meta-analysis of 19 studies revealed that exposure to second hand smoke increased the risk of ischemic heart disease by 30%.[4] A subsequent epidemiological review confirmed that nonsmokers exposed to environmental smoke had a 25% increased risk of coronary heart disease as compared with nonsmokers not exposed to smoke.[5]

- In a meta-analysis of 17 studies (10 from North America, 6 from Europe and 1 from Australasia) researchers concluded that there was a 10% reduction in the incidence of acute coronary events following the introduction of smoke-free legislation.[6]

- Second hand smoke also raises the risk of sustaining a stroke by 30%. This was noted in an analysis of 21,743 participants, aged 45 or older, in the Reasons for Geographic and Racial Differences in Stroke study. No association was sound between second hand smoke exposure and hemorrhagic stroke.[7]

- According to the Centers for Disease Control and Prevention, since 1964, exposure to second hand smoke has resulted in approximately 2,500,000 deaths in nonsmokers from health problems. This includes several cardiovascular deaths.[8]

Conclusion

Second hand smoke is detrimental to the respiratory and cardiovascular health of the innocent inhalers. It is responsible for at least 35,000 deaths annually in the United States. Due to increasing prohibition of indoor public smoking, the home is now becoming the primary source of tobacco second hand smoke exposure,[9] with almost 40% of the children worldwide being exposed to these harmful toxins in their own homes.

Lifestyle Implications

Second hand smoke is harmful. Stay away from people who smoke.

References

1. Lofroth G. Environmental tobacco smoke: overview of chemical composition and Genotoxic components. Mutat Res 1989;222:73–80.
2. Oberg M., Jaakkola M. S., Woodward A., Peruga A., Prüss-Ustün A. 2011 Worldwide burden of disease from exposure to second-hand smoke: A retrospective analysis of data from 192 countries. Lancet, 377, 139–146
3. Lightwood J. M., Glantz S. A. (2009). Declines in acute myocardial infarction after smoke-free laws and individual risk attributable to secondhand smoke. Circulation, 120, 1373–1379
4. Law MR, Morris JK, Wald NJ. Environmental tobacco smoke exposure and ischaemic heart disease: An evaluation of the evidence. BMJ. 1997;315:973–80.
5. He J, Vupputuri S, Allen K, Prerost MR, Hughes J, Whelton PK. Passive smoking and the risk of coronary heart disease – a meta-analysis of epidemiologic studies. N Engl J Med. 1999;340:920–6.
6. Mackay D. F., Irfan M. O., Haw S., Pell J. P. (2010). Meta-analysis of the effect of comprehensive smoke-free legislation on acute coronary events. Heart, 96, 1525–1530
7. Angela M. Malek, Angela M. Malek, Mary Cushman, Daniel T. Lackland, George Howard, Leslie A. McClure, Secondhand Smoke Exposure and Stroke. AJPM. December 2015 Volume 49, Issue 6, Pages e89–e97.
8. U.S. Department of Health and Human Services. The Health Consequences of Smoking—50 Years of Progress: A Report of the Surgeon General. Atlanta: U.S. Department of Health and Human Services, Centers for Disease Control and Prevention, National Center for Chronic Disease Prevention and Health Promotion, Office on Smoking and Health, 2014.
9. Van Deusen A., Hyland A., Travers M.J., Wang C., Higbee C., King B.A., Alford T., Cummings K.M. Secondhand smoke and particulate matter exposure in the home. Nic. Tob. Res. 2009;11:635–641.

70. SHELLFISH

Introduction

Shell fish has been used as a food for hundreds of thousands of years. They include marine molluscs such as clams, mussels, oysters, winkles, and scallops; crustaceans such as shrimp, lobsters, crayfish, and crabs and echinoderms such as sea urchin roe. These are usually of salt-water origin but occasionally freshwater crayfish and river mussels are also called "shellfish". Shell fish are high in cholesterol and hence often considered as bad for the cardiovascular system. A 100-gram serving of clams or mussels has less than 40 milligrams of cholesterol. Scallops contain 30 to 40 milligrams of cholesterol per 100-gram portion, while oysters, provide less than 50 milligrams of cholesterol per 100 grams. However, most studies have failed to connect shellfish consumption with adverse cardiovascular outcomes. Shellfish, in addition to having lower overall fat and saturated fat than other meats, contain high-quality protein and are good sources of omega 3 fatty acids, iron, zinc, copper, and vitamin B-12.

Scientific Evidence

- In a study of 18,244 men aged 45-64 years in Shanghai, China, researchers found that weekly fish/shellfish intake resulted in an approximately 20% reduction in total mortality from coronary heart disease.[1]
- An inverse association between fish and shellfish intake and the occurance of type 2 diabetes in women was also noted in a prospective population-based cohort study in 51,963 men and 64,193 women, initially free of type 2 diabetes, in China.[2]
- There does not seem to be any major published data on shellfish consumption and stroke. However, findings in the coronary artery disease study, can suggest that if there is a relationship, it probably would be a beneficial one.

Conclusion

Shellfish is popular as food. Although high in cholesterol, they have less saturated fat than other meats. They are also a good source of the beneficial omega 3 fatty acids. They are low in calories – for example, crab meat contains only 128 calories in 100g. Scientific data has failed to demonstrate any detrimental cardiovascular effects from eating shellfish.

Lifestyle Implications

Eat shellfish without having any concerns of damaging your cardiovascular system.

References

1. Yuan JM, Ross RK, Gao YT, Yu MC. Fish and shellfish consumption in relation to death from myocardial infarction among men in Shanghai, China. Am J Epidemiol. 2001 Nov 1;154(9):809-16.
2. Raquel Villegas, Yong-Bing Xiang, Tom Elasy, et al. Fish, shellfish, and long-chain n−3 fatty acid consumption and risk of incident type 2 diabetes in middle-aged Chinese men and women. Am J Clin Nutr August 2011. vol. 94 no. 2 543-551

71. SHIFT WORK (AND NIGHT WORK)

Introduction

Shift and night work is common throughout the world. It is designed to provide services usually around the clock - 24/7. It is estimated that globally, 15%-30% of workers do shift work.[1] Shift work including night work has been known to be associated with an increased incidence of several chronic diseases including the metabolic syndrome, diabetes, peptic ulcers, mental health problems, breast cancer and many other cancers.[2] It has also been implicated as a risk factor for cardiovascular diseases.[3]

Scientific Evidence

- There was more hypertension in a study of 1,838 female workers doing shift night work.[4] In another study, there were more hypertension diagnosed individuals in the night workers (6.9%) than in the non-night worker group. (4.6%).[5]
- There are behavioral changes related to night shift work such as increased smoking and a higher risk of developing obesity.[6]
- There is an increased incidence of metabolic syndrome and diabetes mellitus.[7]
- Shift work results in circadian rhythm disruption which contributes to the development of cardiovascular disease.[8] Circadian misalignment-mediated changes increase inflammation – a major factor contributing to atherosclerosis.[9]
- There is also a negative impact from deleterious psychosocial mechanisms generated by difficulties in controlling working hours, decreased work - life balance, insufficient sleep, poor recovery following work and increased social stress.[10] These contribute to the development of atherosclerosis in the night shift workers.[11]
- Women working night and evening shifts have increased all-cause mortality, including that due to cardiovascular diseases, diabetes, Alzheimer's disease and dementia.[7]
- In a large meta-analysis, shift workers were found to have a 24% elevated coronary heart disease risk when compared to non-shift workers.[12]

Conclusion

Scientific data is clear that shift work, including night shift work is detrimental for human health, and especially to the cardiovascular health. Shift workers have higher cardiovascular risk factors, including hypertension, metabolic syndrome, diabetes mellitus, obesity, smoking and psycho-social maladjustments. They exhibit an increased cardiovascular morbidity and mortality.

Lifestyle Implications.

Shift work and night shift work, may have a negative effect on your cardiovascular health.

References

1. Bureau of Labor Statistics US (2005) Workers on Flexible and Shift Schedules in May2004 (US Department of Labor, Washington, DC.
2. Wang X, Armstrong M, Cairns B, Key T, Travis R. Shift work and chronic disease: the epidemiological evidence. Occup Med. 2011;61:78–89.
3. Céline Vetter, Elizabeth E. Devore, Lani R. Wegrzyn, et al. Association between rotating night shift work and risk of coronary heart disease among women. AMA. 2016 April 26; 315(16): 1726–1734.
4. Chen JD, Lin YC, Hsiao ST. Obesity and high blood pressure of 12-hour night shift female clean-room workers. Chronobiol Int. 2010;27:334–44.
5. Park S, Nam J, Lee J-K, Oh S-S, Kang H-T, Koh S-B. Association between night work and cardiovascular diseases: analysis of the 3rd Korean working conditions survey. Annals of Occupational and Environmental Medicine. 2015;27:15.
6. Nabe-Nielsen K, Garde AH, Tüchsen F, Hogh A, Diderichsen F. Cardiovascular risk factors and primary selection into shift work. Scand J Work Environ Health 2008;34(3):206-212.
7. Jørgensen JT, Karlsen S, Stayner L, Hansen J, Andersen ZJ. Shift work and overall and cause-specific mortality in the Danish nurse cohort. Scand J Work Environ Health 2017;43(2):117-126.
8. Frost P, Kolstad HA, Bonde JP. Shift work and the risk of ischemic heart disease—a systematic review of the epidemiologic evidence. Scand J Work Environ Health. 2009;35:163–179.
9. Christopher J. Morrisa, Taylor E, et al. Circadian misalignment increases cardiovascular disease risk factors in humans. PNAS. February 8, 2016.
10. Harrington JM. Health effects of shift work and extended hours of work. Occup Environ Med.2001; 58(1):68–72.
11. S. Jankowiak, E. Backé, F. Liebers, et al. Current and cumulative night shift work and subclinical atherosclerosis: results of the Gutenberg Health Study. Int Arch Occup Environ Health (2016) 89:1169–1182.

12. Vyas MV, Garg AX, Iansavichus AV, et al. Shift work and vascular events: systematic review and meta-analysis. BMJ. 2012; 345: e4800.

72. SITTING

Introduction

Americans on an average sit about 8 hours per day.[1] Excessive sitting is a sedentary behavior that is a risk factor for cardiovascular disease. Activities such as sitting, lying down, watching television, writing and reading, do not increase energy expenditure above the resting level of 1.0–1.5 METs (metabolic equivalents) and are considered as sedentary behaviour. Physical inactivity or sedentary behavior is estimated to result in a 9% premature mortality worldwide. Excessive leisure time sitting increases the risk of several diseases, such as obesity, diabetes and cancer. It increases premature death from all causes. It also increases cardiovascular diseases,[2] and cardiovascular mortality.[3]

Scientific Evidence

- Sitting increases obesity.[4] The disturbing increases in juvenile obesity have received a great deal of attention in the scientific and popular press and have been attributed partly to television viewing, computer games and other sedentary behaviors. These behaviours compete with activities that would have involved physical activity.

- Uninterrupted long periods of sitting may increase hyperglycemia. A recent randomized clinical trial (Diabetes Prevention Program) showed that an intensive lifestyle modification (healthy diet and moderate physical activity of 30 minutes a day for 5 days a week) reduced the incidence of type 2 diabetes by 50% as compared with placebo.[5]

- Inactivity worsens several cardiovascular risk factors,[6] including high-density lipoprotein cholesterol levels, adiposity, fasting glucose levels, type 2 diabetes control, and blood pressure. These risk factors greatly affect cardiovascular health. Sitting also worsens endothelial function.

- Sitting increases cardiovascular diseases.[6] In the NIH-AARP study, when 240,819 US participants, aged 50–71 years, were monitored for 8.5 years, sedentary time was found to be directly related to cardiovascular mortality.[7] In a retrospective study of 5,159 men aged 40 to 59 years and with no history of coronary heart disease and followed for 16.8 years, physical activity was inversely related to coronary heart disease.[8] On the other hand, increased physical activity has been associated with a reduced risk for cardiovascular disease in the general population. Prolonged sitting times also increases cardiovascular mortality.

Conclusion

Sedentary activity is dangerous for the health - staying physically active is good for your health. The Center for Disease Control and Prevention advices the general population to partake in, "activity that, when added to baseline activity, produces health benefits. Brisk walking, jumping rope, dancing, playing tennis or soccer, lifting weights, climbing on playground equipment at recess, and doing yoga are all examples of health-enhancing physical activity." The American Heart Association also recommends physical activity incorporating 150 minutes per week of moderate exercise (thirty minutes a day five times a week) or 75 minutes per week of vigorous exercise (or a combination of moderate and vigorous activity) for cardiovascular health benefits.[9]

Lifestyle Implications

Sit less each day, reduce your total sitting time and you will live healthier and live longer.

References

1. Matthews CE, Chen KY, Freedson PS, Buchowski MS, Beech BM, Pate RR, Troiano RP: Amount of time spent in sedentary behaviors in the United States, 2003–2004. Am J Epidemiol 2008, 167(7):875–881.
2. Stamatakis E, Hamer M, Dunstan DW. Screen-based entertainment time, all-cause mortality, and cardiovascular events: population-based study with ongoing mortality and hospital events follow-up. J Am Coll Cardiol 2011;57:292–99.
3. Kim Y, Wilkens LR, Park SY, Goodman MT, Monroe KR, Kolonel LN. Association between various sedentary behaviours and all-cause, cardiovascular disease and cancer mortality: the Multiethnic Cohort Study. Int J Epidemiol. 2013;42:1040–56.
4. Hu FB. Sedentary lifestyle and risk of obesity and type 2 diabetes. Lipids. 2003 Feb;38(2):103-8.
5. Knowler WC, Barrett-Connor E, Fowler SC, et al. Reduction in the incidence of type 2 diabetes with lifestyle intervention or metformin. N Engl J Med. 2002;346(6):393–403.

6. Ford ES, Caspersen CJ. Sedentary behaviour and cardiovascular disease: a review of prospective studies. International journal of epidemiology. 2012;41(5):1338-1353.

7. Matthews CE, George SM, Moore SC, et al. Amount of time spent in sedentary behaviors and cause-specific mortality in US adults. Am J Clin Nutr. 2012;95:437– 445.

8. Wannamethee SG, Shaper AG, Alberti KG. Physical activity, metabolic factors, and the incidence of coronary heart disease and type 2 diabetes. Arch Intern Med. 2000 Jul 24;160(14):2108-16.

9. http://www.heart.org/HEARTORG/HealthyLiving/PhysicalActivity/Fit nessBasics/American-Heart-Association-Recommendations-for-Physical-Activity-in-Adults_UCM_307976_Article.jsp#.WRKU2uXys1I (Accessed May 8, 2017)

73. SLEEP

Introduction

Adequate sleep is necessary for good health and survival. The amount of sleep each person needs each day depends on many factors, including age. Adults average about 7- 8 hours of sleep per day. Women in the first 3 months of pregnancy and infants generally require more sleep than usual. Several theories have been advanced to explain the function of sleep and include conserving caloric expenditures, replenishing brain energy stores, removing toxic byproducts generated during waking, and nervous system recuperation including connectivity and plasticity functions. Unfortunately, sleep deprivation is becoming more prevalent all over the world. Sleep insufficiency is associated with a plethora of health problems.[1] Inadequate sleep increases insulin resistance, carbohydrate craving, increased caloric consumption, and may increase the risk of developing diabetes. The immune system is compromised and there is an increases susceptibility to infection. Sleepiness is also responsible for many car accidents and fatalities. Chronic inadequate sleep is also related to a higher all-cause mortality. Habitually short sleep durations are associated with increased hypertension. There is also an increase in cardiovascular morbidity and mortality.[2]

Scientific Evidence

- Sleep deprivation is closely connected with an increased incidence of hypertension. Individuals sleeping less than 6 hours/night are 20–32% more likely to develop hypertension compared to those sleeping 7–8 hours.[3] Inadequate sleep deprivation is also related to an attenuated nocturnal dipping in blood pressure, which prognosticates cardiovascular disease.
- Several studies have documented that short sleep hours increase the risk of getting type 2 diabetes.[4] Sleep deprivation also raises the incidence of obesity.[5]
- Sleep deprivation is also associated with an increased rate of coronary artery calcification. Coronary artery calcification prognosticates future cardiovascular events. Compared to 7–8 hours/night, self-reported sleep of ≤5 hours were associated with a

25% raised risk for coronary heart disease in a large study of postmenopausal women.[6]

- Sleep deprivation is associated with increased inflammation, increased sympathetic activity and higher cortisol levels in healthy subjects.[7]

- Short sleep duration is also associated with an increased risk of stroke.[8] A study of 93,175 postmenopausal women found that both self-reported short (≤6 hours/night) sleep duration was significantly associated with ischemic stroke, (including fatal and non-fatal events) during a 7.5-year follow-up.[9]

Conclusion

Sleep is necessary in adequate quatintiy and of good quality for proper health. Observational and experimental data continue to confirm the close association between inadequate sleep and significant health ill effects including excess propensity to develop cardiovascular diseases and increase cardiovascular mortality.

Lifestyle Implications

Sleep well, with adequate quality and quantity.

References

1. Institute of Medicine. Sleep disorders and sleep deprivation: An unmet public health problem. Washington, D.C.: National Academies Press; 2006.
2. King CR, Knutson KL, Rathouz PJ, et al. Short sleep duration and incident coronary artery calcification. JAMA 2008;300(24):2859-2866.
3. Guo XF, Zheng LQ, Wang J, et al. Epidemiological evidence for the link between sleep duration and high blood pressure: a systematic review and meta-analysis. Sleep Med. 2013; 14(4):324–32.
4. Cappuccio FP, D'Elia L, Strazzullo P, Miller MA. Quantity and quality of sleep and incidence of type 2 diabetes: a systematic review and meta-analysis. Diabetes Care. 2010;33:414–20.
5. Knutson KL, Van Cauter E. Associations between sleep loss and increased risk of obesity and diabetes. Ann NY Acad Sci. 2008;1129:287–304.
6. Sands-Lincoln M, Loucks EB, Lu B, et al. Sleep duration, insomnia, and coronary heart disease among postmenopausal women in the Women's Health Initiative. J Womens Health. 2013; 22(6): 477–86.

7. Knutson KL, Spiegel K, Penev P, Van Cauter E: The metabolic consequences of sleep deprivation. Sleep medicine reviews, 2007; 11: 163-178.

8. Ge BH, Guo XM. Short and long sleep durations are both associated with increased risk of stroke: a meta-analysis of observational studies. Int J Stroke. 2015; 10(2):177–84.

9. Chen JC, Brunner RL, Ren H, et al. Sleep duration and risk of ischemic stroke in postmenopausal women. Stroke. 2008; 39(12):3185–92.

74. SMOKING

Introduction

Smoking involves burning the dried leaves of the tobacco plant, rolled into a cigarette, and inhaling the resulting smoke. This activity dates as far back as 5000 BCE. Tobacco smoke is a complex mixture of over 5,000 identified chemicals, many of them toxic and carcinogenic. The main active compound is a para-sympathomimetic stimulant and an alkaloid, called nicotine. Nicotine is a stimulant and highly addictive. Smoking is associated with a plethora of deleterious health conditions, including chronic obstructive pulmonary disease, lung and other cancers, diabetes mellitus, dental ailments, rheumatoid arthritis and cataracts. It also affects men's fertility and can cause significant problems during pregnancy. It is responsible for more than 480,000 deaths each year in the United States. Smoking is also a major and independent risk factor for cardiovascular disease, including atherosclerotic vascular disease, hypertension, myocardial infarction, unstable angina, sudden cardiac death, and stroke.[1] Smoking increases the risk of coronary heart disease and stroke by 2 to 4 times. According to an epidemiological study >1 in 10 cardiovascular deaths, which make up 54% of all deaths worldwide, are related to smoking.[2]

Scientific Evidence

- Blood pressure and heart rate increase during smoking, due to the effects of nicotine. Long term, the effects of smoking on blood pressure are equivocal. However, hypertensives who smoke are more likely to be resistant to treatment.[3]
- Cigarette smoking causes impairment of endothelial function, arterial stiffness, inflammation, and other changes that lead to the initiation, and acceleration of the atherothrombotic process. Atherosclerosis is the main driver of major cardiovascular events.[4]
- In a case-control study of acute myocardial infarction, done in 52 countries, investigators enrolled 15,152 cases and 14,820 controls. They found that smokers had more than double the risk of getting a heart attack.[5] Smokers who quit gain a substantial benefit in the form of decreased coronary heart disease mortality compared to those who continue to smoke

- Similarly, smoking more than doubles the risk of developing a stroke. Quitting smoking results in a rapid decrease in the risk for ischemic stroke.[6]

- Active smoking is associated with significantly increased risks of total mortality.[7] Cessation of smoking reverses this trend. Quitting smoking leads to an improved survival compared to those who continue to smoke.[8]

- Smoking has many deleterious cardiovascular effects including endothelial dysfunction, increased arterial stiffness, increased oxidative stress, and decreased nitric oxide bioavailability, besides others. These harmful effects initiate and accelerate atherosclerosis leading to the higher cardiovascular morbidity and mortality in smokers.

Conclusion

Smoking is a popular activity all over the world. It is also deadly. It is estimated that male smokers lose an average of 13.2 years of life and female smokers lose an average of 14.5 years of life, because of cigarette smoking. The negative impact on the cardiovascular system is significant, including a 2-4 times risk of getting a heart attack or stroke. These odds improve upon quitting. Smoking cessation aids and programs are available all over the country.

Lifestyle Implications

Do not smoke. If you are already a smoker — the best lifestyle decision you can make is to stop smoking.

References

1. Ambrose JA, Barua RS. The pathophysiology of cigarette smoking and cardiovascular disease: an update. J Am Coll Cardiol 43: 1731–1737, 2004; White WB. Smoking-related morbidity and mortality in the cardiovascular setting. Prev Cardiol 10, Suppl 2: 1–4, 2007.

2. Ezzati M, Henley SJ, Thun MJ, Lopez AD. Role of smoking in global and regional cardiovascular mortality. Circulation 112: 489–497, 2005.

3. Khalili P, Nilsson PM, Nilsson JA, Berglund G. Smoking as a modifier of the systolic blood pressure-induced risk of cardiovascular events and mortality: a population-based prospective study of middle-aged men. J Hypertens 20: 1759–1764, 2002.

4. Howard G, Wagenknecht LE, Burke GL, Diez-Roux A, Evans GW, McGovern P, Nieto FJ, Tell GS. Cigarette smoking and progression of atherosclerosis: the Atherosclerosis Risk in Communities (ARIC) study. JAMA 279: 119–124, 1998.

5. Teo KK, Ounpuu S, Hawken Set al. INTERHEART Study Investigators Tobacco use and risk of myocardial infarction in 52 countries in the INTERHEART study: a case-control study. Lancet 368: 647–658, 2006.

6. Ockene IS, Miller NH. Cigarette smoking, cardiovascular disease, and stroke: a statement for healthcare professionals from the American Heart Association. American Heart Association Task Force on Risk Reduction. Circulation 96: 3243–3247, 1997.

7. Pan A, Wang Y, Talaei M, Hu FB. Relation of Smoking with Total Mortality and Cardiovascular Events Among Patients with Diabetes: A Meta-Analysis and Systematic Review. Circulation. 2015;132(19):1795-1804.

8. Salonen JT. Stopping smoking and long-term mortality after acute myocardial infarction. Br Heart J. 1980;43:463-469.

75. SODA/SUGAR SWEETENED BEVERAGES

Introduction

Carbonated beverages were developed in the 1760's and sugar was not added to these popular drinks. Today, sugar sweetened beverages are available everywhere and are routinely consumed. Unfortunately, these sodas/beverages increase the risk of diabetes mellitus, coronary artery disease and strokes. Despite this, the consumption of sugar-sweetened beverages, including sodas, vitamin water, and energy drinks, continues to be high in the United States. In 2009, per capita consumption of these drinks was estimated at 45 gallons/year. This accounted for nearly half of the total beverage intake.[1] Although the soda consumption in the United States may be declining, according to the Centers for Disease Control and Prevention, in 2011-2014, 63% of the youth and 49% of the adults still drank a sugar-sweetened beverage on a given day.[2]

Scientific Evidence

- In a review done in 2010, Malik and associates highlighted the increased propensity to develop obesity, type 2 diabetes and cardiovascular disease with the intake of sugar sweetened beverages.[3]
- In an analysis of 40,389 healthy men from the Health Professionals Follow-Up Study, during a 20-year monitoring period, a causal link was noted between soda intake and diabetes mellitus. Sugar sweetened beverage drinkers had a 24% higher risk of developing diabetes mellitus.[4] In this study, the risk of developing diabetes mellitus fell by 17% if one serving of sugar-sweetened beverage was replaced with 1 cup of coffee.
- In the Nurses' Health Study, a positive association between sugar sweetened beverage intake and risk of coronary heart disease (nonfatal myocardial infarction or fatal coronary heat disease) was observed in over 88,000 women followed for 24 years. Nurses who consumed $\geq$ 2 sugar sweetened beverages per day had a 35% greater risk of developing coronary heart disease compared to those who consumed <1 sugar sweetened beverages per month.[5]
- Soda intake is also associated with a higher risk of stroke. This conclusion was gleaned from the Nurses' Health Study (a

prospective cohort study of 84,085 women followed for 28 years), and the Health Professionals Follow-Up Study (a prospective cohort study of 43,371 men followed for 22 years). There were 1,416 strokes in men during the 841,770 person-years of follow-up and 2,938 strokes in women during 2,188,230 person-years of follow-up. Greater drinkers of sugar-sweetened and low-calorie sodas experienced a 16% higher risk of stroke. [6]

- Mechanisms for this cardiovascular damage include hyperglycemia, dyslipidemia, inflammation, or endothelial dysfunction.[7]

Conclusion

The 2010 Dietary Guidelines provide a specific limit for discretionary calories, (those from added sugars, additional fats, and alcohol) and recommend that their total intake be limited to 5--15% of total energys.[8] However, many Americans continue to exceed these dietary 'added sugar' recommendations.[9] A large amount of blame is to be assigned to sugar sweetened beverages. The increased intake of sugar sweetened beverages elevates the risk of diabetes mellitus, coronary artery disease and strokes.

Lifestyle Implications

Stay away from soda and other sugar sweetened beverages. Substitute them with other beverages, like coffee, tea or the best drink of all - water.

References

1. Andreyeva T, Chaloupka FJ, Brownell KD. Estimating the potential of taxes on sugar-sweetened beverages to reduce consumption and generate revenue. Prev Med 2011;52:413–6.
2. Welsh JA, Sharma AJ, Grellinger L, Vos MB. Consumption of added sugars is decreasing in the United States. Am J Clin Nutr 2011;94:726–34. https://www.cdc.gov/nutrition/data-statistics/sugar-sweetened-beverages-intake.html
3. Malik VS, Popkin BM, Bray GA, Despres JP, Hu FB. Sugar-sweetened beverages, obesity, type 2 diabetes mellitus, and cardiovascular disease risk. Circulation 2010;121:1356–64.
4. de Koning L, Malik VS, Rimm EB, Willett WC, Hu FB. Sugar-sweetened and artificially sweetened beverage consumption and risk of type 2 diabetes in men. Am J Clin Nutr 2011;93:1321–7.
5. Fung TT, Malik V, Rexrode KM, Manson JE, Willett WC, Hu FB. Sweetened beverage consumption and risk of coronary heart disease in women. Am J Clin Nutr 2009;89:1037 - 42

6. Bernstein AM, De Koning L, Flint AJ, Rexrode KM, Willett WC. Soda consumption and the risk of stroke in men and women. Am J Clin Nutr 2012;95:1190–9.

7. Fung TT, Malik V, Rexrode KM, Manson JE, Willett WC, Hu FB. Sweetened beverage consumption and risk of coronary heart disease in women. Am J Clin Nutr 2009;89:1037 - 42.

8. US Department of Agriculture US dietary guidelines for Americans, 2010. Available from: http://www.cnpp.usda.gov/dietaryguidelines.htm.

9. Welsh JA, Sharma AJ, Grellinger L, Vos MB. Consumption of added sugars is decreasing in the United States. The American Journal of Clinical Nutrition. 2011;94(3):726-734.

76. SOCIALIZING

Introduction

Loneliness is a major social and public health problem, worldwide. Almost 32% of adults over the age of 55 report loneliness, with 5-7% reporting the feelings as being intense or persistent. Loneliness or social isolation plays an important role in health and longevity. Lonely or socially isolated adults are at an increased risk of several health problems and premature mortality. A large study found that lack of socialization and social relationships increased the risk of stroke and coronary heart disease by about 30%.[1] It is also associated with premature cardiovascular mortality.[2]

Scientific Evidence

- There is an improvement in depression following interventions promoting active social contact and creativity in a population over 65 years of age.[3] Depression is a significant risk factor for cardiovascular disease.
- Social isolation or loneliness increases the blood pressure.[4]
- In a large meta-analysis of 23 scientific papers, loneliness or social isolation was associated with an increase in coronary heart disease and stroke.[1]
- Social interactions improve physical activity, while loneliness tends to decrease it. The latter also encourages discontinuation of an ongoing activity. Social interactions also impact obesity. Lonely people are less likely to walk for leisure or transportation, which would help them lose weight.[5]
- Loneliness increases smoking, a major risk factor for cardiovascular diseases. Socialization may involve mild to moderate alcohol drinking, and moderate alcohol intake has beneficial effects on the heart.
- Loneliness increases systemic and vascular inflammation.[6] In animal studies involving prairie voles, animals that have similar social interactions as humans, social isolation produced depressive behaviors, increased heart rate, heart rhythm dysregulation, and autonomic imbalance due to increased sympathetic and decreased parasympathetic drive to the heart.
- Loneliness increases premature mortality.[7]

Conclusion

Loneliness and social isolation initiates a cascade of harmful changes that lead to premature cardiovascular disease and premature cardiovascular death. This has been documented in several animals, epidemiological and clinical studies. Lack of social relationships is associated with an increased risk of developing coronary heart disease and stroke of around 30%.[1]

Lifestyle Implications.

Loneliness is associated with poor health behaviors and an increased morbidity and premature mortality. Get socially active.

References

1. Valtorta NK, Kanaan M, Gilbody S, Ronzi S, Hanratty B. Loneliness and social isolation as risk factors for coronary heart disease and stroke: systematic review and meta-analysis of longitudinal observational studies. Heart. 2016;102(13):1009-1016.
2. Penninx BW, van Tilburg T, Kriegsman DM, Deeg DJ, Boeke AJ, van Eijk JT. Effects of social support and personal coping resources on mortality in older age: The Longitudinal Aging Study Amsterdam. American Journal of Epidemiology. 1997;146(6):510–519.
3. Greaves CJ, Farbus L. Effects of creative and social activity on the health and well-being of socially isolated older people: outcomes from a multi-method observational study. J R Soc Promot Health. 2006 May;126(3):134-42.
4. Hawkley LC, Masi CM, Berry JD, Cacioppo JT. Loneliness is a unique predictor of age-related differences in systolic blood pressure. Psychology and Aging. 2006;21(1):152–164.
5. Lauder W, Mummery K, Jones M, Caperchione C. A comparison of health behaviours in lonely and non-lonely populations. Psychology Health & Medicine. 2006;11:233–245.
6. Cole SW, Hawkley LC, Arevalo JM, Sung CY, Rose RM, Cacioppo JT. Social regulation of gene expression in human leukocytes. Genome Biology. 2007;8(9): R189.181–R189.113. PMCID: PMC2375027.
7. Penninx BW, van Tilburg T, Kriegsman DM, Deeg DJ, Boeke AJ, van Eijk JT. Effects of social support and personal coping resources on mortality in older age: The Longitudinal Aging Study Amsterdam. American Journal of Epidemiology. 1997;146(6):510–519.

77. SPORTS

Introduction

Sports activity has been regularly recommended by physicians of the ancient and modern world – for staying healthy. Evidence based data from several scientific studies and meta-analyses persuasively confirm a positive association between increased athletic activity (both recreational and competitive) and enhanced cardiovascular health.[1] Competitive endurance athletes enjoy a longer life span (primarily due to a lower cardiovascular mortality) than the general population.[2] Strength-based sports, on the other hand, do not seem to impart the same benefit. Regular aerobic athletic activity improves the cardiac reserve.[3] Recreational sports may also be a good way of complying with the American Heart Association exercise recommendations.[4]

Scientific Evidence

- There are benefits of regular exercise that are also seen in people playing recreational or competitive sports. These include a reduction in blood pressure,[5] improvement in the lipid profile,[6] reduction of abdominal adiposity,[7] improved insulin sensitivity, better glucose metabolism,[8] reduced systemic inflammation,[9] and improvement in overall cardio-vascular function.[10]
- Participants in sports activity are more likely to have cardiovascular healthy lifestyle behaviors.[11]
- Sports activity involves social interactions and generates several positive emotions such as enthusiasm and optimism, factors that help improve many psychological risk factors (stress, anxiety and depression), that are otherwise detrimental for cardiovascular diseases.[12]
- Competitive endurance athletes enjoy a longer life span (primarily due to a lower cardiovascular mortality) than the general population.[13]

Conclusion

The American Heart Association recommends at least 150 minutes per week of moderate exercise (thirty minutes a day five times a week) or 75 minutes per week of vigorous exercise (or a combination of moderate and vigorous activity) for cardiovascular health benefits. Playing active sports should help meet these recommendations for exercise, besides providing other cardiovascular benefits. A word of caution - sports activities can cause different injuries, from joint to head injuries.[14] Also if you have health problems, participation in certain sports may be contraindicated.[15]

Lifestyle Implications

Playing recreational (and competitive) sports is a good method of cardiovascular health promotion.

References

1. Haskell, W. L., Lee, I-M., Pate, R. R., et al. (2007). Physical activity and public health: Updated recommendation for adults from the American College of Sports Medicine and the American Heart Association. Circulation, Volume 116, Issue 9, 2007, pages 1081-1093.
2. Teramoto M, Bungum TJ: Mortality and longevity of elite athletes. J Sci Med Sport 2010; 13: 410–6.
3. Jürgen Scharhag, Herbert Löllgen, Wilfried Kindermann. Competitive Sports and the Heart: Benefit or Risk? Deutsches Ärzteblatt International. Dtsch Arztebl Int 2013; 110(1–2): 14–24.
4. http://www.heart.org/HEARTORG/HealthyLiving/PhysicalActivity/FitnessBasics/American-Heart-Association-Recommendations-for-Physical-Activity-in-Adults_UCM_307976_Article.jsp#.WRCeLeXys1I. accessed May 8, 2017.
5. Blair SN, Goodyear NN, Gibbons LW, et al. Physical fitness and incidence of hypertension in healthy normotensive men and women. JAMA 1984;252:487-90.
6. Berg A, Halle M, Franz I, et al. Physical activity and lipoprotein metabolism: epidemiological evidence and clinical trials. Eur J Med Res 1997;2:259-64.
7. Tremblay A, Despres JP, Leblanc C, et al. Effect of intensity of physical activity on body fatness and fat distribution. Am J Clin Nutr 1990;51:153-7.
8. Wallberg-Henriksson H, Rincon J, Zierath JR. Exercise in the management of non-insulin-dependent diabetes mellitus. Sports Med 1998;25:25-35.
9. Adamopoulos S, Parissis J, Kroupis C, et al. Physical training reduces peripheral markers of inflammation in patients with chronic heart failure. Eur Heart J 2001;22:791-7.

10. Warburton DE, Haykowsky MJ, Quinney HA, et al. Blood volume expansion and cardiorespiratory function: effects of training modality. Med Sci Sports Exerc 2004;36:991-1000.

11. Pate RR, Trost SG, Levin S, Dowda M. Sports participation and health-related behaviors among US youth. Arch Pediatr Adolesc Med. 2000 Sep;154(9):904-11.

12. Dunn AL, Trivedi MH, O'Neal HA. Physical activity dose–response effects on outcomes of depression and anxiety. [discussion 609-10]. Med Sci Sports Exerc 2001;33:S587-97.

13. Teramoto M, Bungum TJ: Mortality and longevity of elite athletes. J Sci Med Sport 2010; 13: 410–6.

14. Radić B, Radić P, Duraković D. Sports and health: equivalence or contrariety. Acta Clin Croat. 2014 Dec;53(4):430-6.

15. Baman TS, Gupta S, Day SM. Cardiovascular Health, Part 2: Sports Participation in Athletes With Cardiovascular Conditions. Sports Health. 2010;2(1):19-28.

Introduction

Dietary supplements are used by more than one half of all Americans, daily or on occasion. Common supplements include vitamins, minerals and herbal products – these are available over the counter without a prescription. They are usually available in a pill, powder or liquid form. Data collected by the National Health and Nutrition Examination Survey from 2003 to 2006 revealed that 33 percent of all adults took multivitamin or multimineral supplements.[1] Other common supplements taken by US residents are fish oil/omega 3/ Docosahexaenoic acid (37.4 percent), glucosamine (19.9 percent), echinacea (19.8 percent), flaxseed oil or pills (15.9 percent), and ginseng (14.1 percent).[2] Some of these 'over the counter' supplements exhibit cardiovascular beneficial effects.

Scientific Evidence

- **Co-enzyme Q10:** This intracellular antioxidant protects the low-density lipoprotein cholesterol from oxidation. It also reduces inflammation. In long term studies, it has been shown to reduce coronary heart disease mortality. The endogenous production of co-enzyme Q10 decreases as age increases.[3] The co-enzyme Q10 concentration has been inversely related to the severity of congestive heart failure, and supplementation with co-enzyme Q10 has been postulated to improve congestive heart failure.[4]

- **Fish Oil:** Eicosapentaenoic acid and docosahexaenoic acid are omega-3 fatty acids that are found in large quantities in fatty fish These have several cardiovascular benefits, including reducing triglyceride levels, reducing inflammation and stabilizing heart rhythm. These cardiovascular benefits have been well documented.[5] However, with the arrival of statins and the widespread use of early revascularization, evidence based benefits of fish oil supplementation for the primary or secondary prevention of coronary heart disease have dwindled.[6]

- **Hawthorn:** This Chinese herb has antioxidant, positive inotropic, anti-inflammatory, and anticardiac remodeling effects. Hawthorn preparations have shown to be beneficial in the treatment of mild to moderate heart failure.[7] They may also have a therapeutic role in the treatment of hypertension, and hyperlipidemia.[8]

- **Psyllium:** Psyllium is a soluble fiber commonly used as a gentle bulk-forming laxative. When psyllium husk comes in contact with water, it swells and forms a gelatin-like-mass. The mass binds bile acids in the intestinal lumen resulting in their decreased absorption and increased fecal excretion, necessitating the liver to use cholesterol to make more bile acids. The result is a lower total cholesterol, as well as a decrease in low-density lipoprotein cholesterol level.[9] The triglyceride and high-density lipoprotein levels may also improve. These lipid actions help psyllium lower the risk of cardiovascular disease.

Conclusion

'Over the counter' supplements are popular. The four heart friendly supplements mentioned here shown evidence based benefits in cardiovascular conditions.

Lifestyle Implications

If these supplements appear to be relevant for you, discuss with your health care provider for clearance to consume them. Psyllium consumption, in particular, is a good way of increasing your fiber intake.

References

1. Bailey RL, Gahche JJ, Lentino CV, et al. Dietary Supplement Use in the United States, 2003–2006. The Journal of Nutrition. 2011;141(2):261-266. doi:10.3945/jn.110.133025.
2. https://nccih.nih.gov/health/supplements/wiseuse.htm
3. Kalen A, Appelkvist EL, Dallner G. Age-related changes in the lipid compositions of rat and human tissues. Lipids. 1989;24(7):579–84. Epub 1989/07/0.
4. Fotino AD, Thompson-Paul AM, Bazzano LA. Effect of coenzyme Q10 supplementation on heart failure: a meta-analysis. The American Journal of Clinical Nutrition. 2013;97(2):268-275.
5. Mozaffarian D, Wu JH. (n-3) fatty acids and cardiovascular health: are effects of EPA and DHA shared or complementary? J Nutr. 2012;142(3):614S–625S.
6. Greene J, Ashburn SM, Razzouk L, Smith DA. Fish Oils, Coronary Heart Disease, and the Environment. American Journal of Public Health. 2013;103(9):1568-1576.

7. Holubarsch CJ, Colucci WS, Meinertz T, Gaus W, Tendera M. The efficacy and safety of Crataegus extract WS 1442 in patients with heart failure: the SPICE trial. Eur J Heart Fail. 2008;10:1255–63.

8. Wang J, Xiong X, Feng B. Effect of Crataegus Usage in Cardiovascular Disease Prevention: An Evidence-Based Approach. Evidence-based Complementary and Alternative Medicine : eCAM. 2013;2013:149363.

9. James W Anderson, Michael H Davidson, Lawrence Blonde, et al. Long-term cholesterol-lowering effects of psyllium as an adjunct to diet therapy in the treatment of hypercholesterolemia. Am J Clin Nutr June 2000 vol. 71 no. 6 1433-1438.

79. SUPPLEMENTS: HEART HARMFUL

Introduction

Some dietary supplements may not only be cardiovascular unsafe but may also interfere with certain medicines or other supplements. They should be avoided.

Scientific Evidence

- **Licorice:** Licorice is a popular sweetener found in many soft drinks, food products, and herbal medicines. Liquorice sweets are popular around the world. Traditionally licorice was used to treat gastric ulcers and sore throat. Taken in excess, licorice root can cause high blood pressure and deplete potassium levels.[1] Low potassium levels can lead to potentially fatal cardiac arrhythmias.[2]

- **Yohimbe:** The bark of the Yohimbe tree (a tall evergreen forest tree native to parts of Africa) is used medicinally. Yohimbine is commonly used in traditional medicine to arouse sexual excitement. It is also touted to improve athletic performance and help with weight loss. It can cause a rapid heart rate and induce high blood pressure. Higher doses, however, may result in a dangerous fall in blood pressure.[3] Yohimbine can interact with blood pressure medications and decrease their effectiveness, especially clonidine.

- **Ephedra:** Ephedra sinica, also known as *ma huang*, is the source of the alkaloid ephedrine. It is commonly used as a supplement to aid weight loss and for nasal decongestion. Dangers of ephedra include high blood pressure, palpitations, stroke and death.[4] Its use in 'over the counter' preperations has been banned by the U.S. Food and Drug Administration.

- **Red Yeast Rice:** Red yeast rice extract, a traditional Chinese medicine, is a substance that is extracted from rice that's been fermented with a yeast called *Monascus purpureus*. Red rice extract and its main active ingredient monacolin K, helps reduce total cholesterol and low-density lipoprotein cholesterol.[5] It should not be used with the 'statin' class of drugs and other cholesterol lowering drugs such as gemfibrozil and fenofibrate. Dangerous side effects include myopathy (muscle damage and weakness) and liver dysfunction. Red yeast rice may also contain a contaminant called citrinin, which can cause kidney failure. The U.S. Food and Drug Administration has banned the sale of red yeast rice products (containing more than trace amounts of monacolin K) as dietary supplements.[6]

Conclusion

Because supplements are regulated as foods, and not as drugs, the Food and Drug Administration doesn't evaluate the quality of supplements or assess their effects on the body. If a product is found to be unsafe after it reaches the market, the Food and Drug Administration can restrict or ban its use. Unfortunately, many people in the U.S. still manage to get ephedra and red yeast rice extract containing products from other countries, often via the internet.

Lifestyle Implications

Dietary supplements do not replace prescription medicines. And they can be unsafe. Do not take products containing ephedra or red rice extract. Let your health provider know of any supplements you take.

References

1. De Klerk G., Nieuwenhuis M., Beutler J. (1997) Hypokalaemia and hypertension associated with use of liquorice flavoured chewing gum. Br Med J 314: 731–732.
2. Miyamoto K., Kawai H., Aoyama R., Watanabe H., Suzuki K., Suga N., et al. (2009) Torsades de Pointes induced by a combination of garenoxacin and disopyramide and other cytochrome P450, family 3, subfamily A polypeptide-4-influencing drugs during hypokalemia due to licorice. Clin Exp Nephrol 14: 164–167.
3. Szabadi E, Bradshaw CM. Autonomic pharmacology of α2-adrenoceptors. J Psychopharmacol. 1996;10:6–18.
4. Haller CA, Benowitz NL. Adverse cardiovascular and central nervous system events associated with dietary supplements containing ephedra alkaloids. N Engl J Med 2000;343:833-8.
5. Li Y, Jiang L, Jia Z, et al. A Meta-Analysis of Red Yeast Rice: An Effective and Relatively Safe Alternative Approach for Dyslipidemia. Calabresi L, ed. PLoS ONE. 2014;9(6): e98611.
6. https://nccih.nih.gov/health/redyeastrice

80. SWIMMING

Introduction

Swimming involves using the arms and legs to move the body through water and is an aerobic activity. As a recreational sport, evidence of its popularity goes back to over 10,000 years - many Stone Age paintings depict swimming. Besides being recreational, it has become popular as a competitive sport. Aerobic exercise is cardiovascular protective. However, many aerobic exercises also involve weight-bearing, and are not suitable for individuals with orthopedic or musculoskeletal limitations, excess adiposity or other medical conditions. Swimming is an attractive alternative for these people to perform and gain the benefits of exercise. Swimming has health benefits comparable to those achieved with walking and running.[1] It is a good exercise for building muscle and endurance. It also helps reduce inflammation and oxidative stress.[2] It is therefore good for the cardiovascular system.[3] Its benefits for cardiovascular protection have been well recorded in the scientific literature.

Scientific Evidence

- In a study of 43 adults older than 50 years, diagnosed with pre-hypertension or mild (stage 1) hypertension, swimming regularly for 15-45 minutes over12 weeks, lowered the systolic blood pressure by 9 mmHg. There was also better arterial elasticity, with the group demonstrating a 21% increase in carotid artery compliance, as well as improvement in flow-mediated dilation and cardiovagal baroreflex sensitivity.[4] These results indicate better health of the arterial vasculature.

- There is a strong association between increased rates of physical activity and increased longevity.[5] Chase and associates studied 40,547 men, aged 20–90 years, during the years 1971–2003. A total of 3,386 deaths occurred during the 543,330 man-years of observation. After adjustment for other risk factors, swimmers had a lower all-cause risk of motality, of 53%, when compared to men who were sedentary, a 50% lower risk when compared to walkers and a 49% lower risk when compared to runners.[6]

- Swimmers have higher cardio-respiratory fitness levels than walkers and sedentary men.[6] Compared to sedentary men, swimmers have lower total cholesterol, triglycerides, fasting blood glucose, and resting heart rates, as well as higher high-density-lipoprotein cholesterol. They also have lower total-cholesterol and triglyceride levels than walkers.

Conclusion

Swimming is one of the few activities that work your whole body. Swimming improves the cardiovascular health profile. It is usually a lifetime activity and can be enjoyed by a large percentage of the general population, including individuals with chronic diseases.[7] However, people who are frail and patients with arthritis, cardiovascular diseases, cancer and type 2 diabetes,[8] should discuss with their health care provider, before embarking on a swimming regimen.

Lifestyle Implications

Swimming is a good cardiovascular exercise, especially if you are unable to do other aerobic and/or weight bearing workouts.

References

1.   Chase, N.L., Sui, X., & Blair, S.N. (2008). Comparison of the health benefits of swimming with other types of physical activity and sedentary lifestyle habits. International Journal of Aquatic Research and Education, 2, 151–161.
2.   Qin L, Yao Z, Chang Q, et al. Swimming attenuates inflammation, oxidative stress, and apoptosis in a rat model of dextran sulfate sodium-induced chronic colitis. Oncotarget. 2017;8(5):7391-7404.
3.   Mohr M, Nordsborg NB, Lindenskov A, et al. High-Intensity Intermittent Swimming Improves Cardiovascular Health Status for Women with Mild Hypertension. BioMed Research International. 2014;2014:728289.
4.   Nualnim N, Parkhurst K, Dhindsa M, Tarumi T, Vavrek J, Tanaka H. Effects of swimming training on blood pressure and vascular function in adults >50 years of age. American Journal of Cardiology. 2012;109(7):1005–1010.
5.   Lee, I.M., & Paffenbarger, R.S., Jr. (2000). Associations of light, moderate, and vigorous intensity physical activity with longevity. The Harvard Alumni Health Study. American Journal of Epidemiology, 151, 293–299.
6.   Nancy L. Chase, Xuemei Sui, and Steven N. Blair. Swimming and All-Cause Mortality Risk Compared With Running, Walking, and Sedentary Habits in Men. International Journal of Aquatic Research and Education, 2008, 2, 213-223.
7.   Westby, M.D. (2001). A health professional's guide to exercise prescription for people with arthritis: A review of aerobic fitness activities. Arthritis and Rheumatism, 45, 501–511.

8.   Sundquist, K., Qvist, J., Sundquist, J., & Johansson, S.E. (2004). Frequent and occasional physical activity in the elderly: A 12-year follow-up study of mortality. American Journal of Preventive Medicine, 27, 22–27.

81. TAI CHI

Introduction

Tai chi (t'ai chi or taiji) originated in China. This technique of martial arts was developed by Wangting Chen towards tthe end of Ming Dynasty (18th century A.D) and is now popular all over the world. It is a gentle physical exercise with slow movements and genrates low impact. It combines physical activity with body awareness, attention to breathing and meditation. Tai chi has been found to have several health benefits, including reducing falls, improving cognitive function and reducing symptoms of arthritis and depression.[1] Benefits have also been reported in improving symptoms and the quality of life in patients with rheumatoid arthritis, human immunodeficiency virus infections, cancer, and heart failure.[2] It can also help reduce fatigue. A considerable amount of scientific work on the benefits of Tai Chi has focused on its ability to reduce blood pressure.[3] Lowering blood pressure plays an important role in decreasing cardiovascular events and death.[4] Tai Chi may also help the cardiovascular system through many other mechanisms.[5]

Scientific Evidence

- Most of the benefits of tai chi have been documented on blood pressure. In a review of twenty-two studies, researchers reported tai chi reduced the systolic blood pressure by 3 - 32 mm Hg and the diastolic blood pressure by 2 -18 mm Hg in hypertensive patients.[6] It also increased exercise capacity.

- Blood pressure lowering effects have also been documented in 1,157 healthy subjects. Blood pressure decreases in these studies ranged from 4 to 18 mm Hg in systolic blood pressure and 2.3 to 7.5 mm Hg in diastolic blood pressure.[3]

- Tai chi improves lipid abnormalities, lowering triglyceride levels.[7] Researchers also found a tendency towards a reduction in total cholesterol levels. Another study reported an improvement in the low-density cholersterol particle size.[8]

- Tai chi practitioners notice weight loss and improvements in metabolic parameters.[9] Tai chi also improves endothelial function.[10]

- Tai chi helps reduce depression and improves general well-being.[11] Depression is associated with cardiovascular disease. It helps improve the quality of life in patients with chronic heart failure.

Conclusion

Tai chi is effective in reducing blood pressure in both healthy and hypertensive subjects. It helps improve the exercise capacity and quality of life in cardiovascular patients. It is safe in patients with coronary artery disease,[12] and in those that are frail.[13]

Lifestyle Implications

Tai Chi is easy and safe to do and helps in reducing blood pressure.

References

1. Michele R. Solloway, Stephanie L. Taylor, et al. An evidence map of the effect of Tai Chi on health outcomes. Systematic Reviews (2016) 5:126.
2. Wang C, Collet JP, Lau J. The effect of Tai Chi on health outcomes in patients with chronic conditions: a systematic review. Arch Intern Med. 2004;164:493–501.
3. Yeh GY, Wang C, Wayne PM, Phillips RS. The effect of tai chi exercise on blood pressure: a systematic review. Prev Cardiol. 2008;11:82–89.
4. Ogden LG, He J, Lydick E, et al. Long-term absolute benefit of lowering blood pressure in hypertensive patients according to the JNC VI risk stratification. Hypertension. 2000;35:539–543.
5. Dalusung-Angosta A. The impact of Tai Chi exercise on coronary heart disease: a systematic review. J Am Acad Nurse Pract. 2011;23(7):376–381.
6. Yeh GY, Wang C, Wayne PM, Phillips R. Tai Chi exercise for patients with cardiovascular conditions and risk factors: a systematic review. J Cardiopulm Rehabil Prev. 2009; 29: 152–160.
7. Xiao-hong Pan, Amina Mahemuti, Xue-hua Zhang, et al. Effect of Tai Chi exercise on blood lipid profiles: a meta-analysis of randomized controlled trials. J Zhejiang Univ Sci B. 2016 Aug; 17(8): 640–648.
8. Beebe N, Magnanti S, Katkowski L, et al. Effects of the addition of t'ai chi to a dietary weight loss program on lipoprotein atherogenicity in obese older women. J Altern Complement Med. 2013;19(9):759–766.
9. Stanley Sai-Chuen Hui, Yao Jie Xie, Jean Woo, and Timothy Chi-Yui Kwok. Effects of Tai Chi and Walking Exercises on Weight Loss, Metabolic Syndrome Parameters, and Bone Mineral Density: A Cluster Randomized Controlled Trial. Evidence-Based Complementary and Alternative Medicine. Volume 2015, Article ID 976123, 10 pages.

10. Frishman WH, Beravol P, Carosella C. Alternative and complementary medicine for preventing and treating cardiovascular disease. Dis Mon. 2009;55(3):121–192.

11. Wang C, Bannuru R, Ramel J, Kupelnick B, Scott T, Schmid CH. Tai Chi on psychological well-being: systematic review and meta-analysis. BMC complement Altern Med. 2010; 10:23.

12. Zheng JQ. The effect of Tai Chi on coronary heart disease rehabilitation in elderly. Chin J Rehabilitation Theory Practice. 2004;10:429.

13. Wolf SL, O'Grady M, Easley KA, et al. The influence of intense Tai Chi training on physical performance and hemodynamic outcomes in transitionally frail, older adults. J Gerontol A Biol Sci Med Sci. 2006;61A:184–189.

82. TEA: BLACK/BROWN

Introduction

Tea is one of the most consumed beverages in the world.[1] Tea is made from the leaves of the evergreen plant, Camellia sinensis.[2] Black tea is made from oxidized tea leaves and accounts for almost 80% of the tea consumed. Originating in China, and called 'chai', black tea is now popular all over the world. China, India, Kenya and Sri Lanka are the largest producers. Tea has many medicinal properties, which has attracted significant medical attention in the recent years.[3] Most of the health benefits have been attributed to the high concentration of several anti-oxidant phenolic compounds in tea.[4] Therapeutic benefits have been noted in cancer, cognitive dysfunction and osteoporosis. More recently, several epidemiological and scientific studies have demonstrated that tea consumption has an inverse relationship with cardiovascular diseases.[5]

Scientific Evidence

- Black tea is rich in phenolic compounds – especially flavonoids. Theaflavins account for 50–60% and catechins 20–30% of total flavonoids in black tea. These polyphenols in tea provide potent anti-oxidant, anti-inflammatory, anti-platelet, anti-vasoconstriction and anti-proliferative effects – all cardioprotective.[6]

- The phenolic compounds present in black tea also help reduce several cardiovascular disease risk factors such as hypertension,[7] diabetes mellitus,[8] dyslipidemia,[9] obesity,[10] stress, anxiety and depression.[11]

- Drinking 3 cups of tea per day decreases the risk of myocardial infarction by 11%.[12]

- In an epidemiological survey of 76,979 Japanese, drinking more than 6 cups of tea per day resulted in reduced cardiovascular disease mortality.[13]

- A 13-year study from Netherlands involving 37,514 healthy adults confirmed the mortality reducing benefits of drinking tea - in this case with a daily intake of 3-6 cups of black tea.[5]

- Tea drinking also reduces strokes by 10%–20%.[14]

Conclusion

Tea drinking is a pleasurable social activity in many parts of the world. Tea drinking also exerts significant cardiovascular benefits. Black tea consumption has repeatedly shown to have an inverse relationship with cardiovascular diseases. The benefits accrue primarily from the phytochemicals, especially catechins and flavonols, abundantly present in the tea leaves. Tea is s popular drink – it is relatively cheap, easy to brew and safe. Drinking tea should be incorporated as a healthy daily lifestyle.

Lifestyle Implications

Tea drinking can be a relaxing social event – and it is good for your heart.

References

1. Weisburger JH. Tea and health: a historical perspective. Cancer Lett. 1997;114(1–2):315–317.
2. Martin, Laura C. (2007). Tea: The Drink that Changed the World. Tuttle Publishing. ISBN 0-8048-3724-4.
3. Chacko SM, Thambi PT, Kuttan R, Nishigaki I. Beneficial effects of green tea: A literature review. Chinese Medicine. 2010;5:13.
4. Balentine DA, Wiseman SA, Bouwens LC. The chemistry of tea flavonoids. Crit Rev Food Sci Nutr. 1997;37 (8):693–704.
5. De Koning Gans JM, Uiterwaal CS, van der Schouw YT, Boer JM, Grobbee DE, Verschuren WM, et al. Tea and coffee consumption and cardiovascular morbidity and mortality. Arterioscler Thromb Vasc Biol. 2010;30:1665–71.
6. Basu A, Lucas EA. Mechanisms and effects of green tea on cardiovascular health. Nutr Rev. 2007 Aug;65(8 Pt 1):361-75.
7. Greyling A, Ras RT, Zock PL, et al. The Effect of Black Tea on Blood Pressure: A Systematic Review with Meta-Analysis of Randomized Controlled Trials. Schillaci G, ed. PLoS ONE. 2014;9(7): e103247.
8. The InterAct Consortium. Tea Consumption and Incidence of Type 2 Diabetes in Europe: The EPIC-InterAct Case-Cohort Study. Herder C, ed. PLoS ONE. 2012;7(5): e36910.
9. Stensvold I, Tverdal A, Solvoll K, Foss OP. Tea consumption. relationship to cholesterol, blood pressure, and coronary and total mortality. Prev Med. 1992;21:546–53.
10. Wu CH, Lu FH, Chang TC, et al. Relationship among habitual tea consumption, percent body fat, and body fat distribution. Obesity. 2003;11(9):1088–1095.
11. Donnelly GF. The tea ceremony: connecting with self and others. Holist Nurs Pract. 2007 Sep-Oct;21(5):215.

12. Peters U, Poole C, Arab L. Does tea affect cardiovascular disease? a meta-analysis. Am J Epidemiol. 2001;154:495–503.

13. Mineharu Y, Koizumi A, Wada Y, et al. Coffee, green tea, black tea and Oolong tea consumption and risk of mortality from cardiovascular disease in Japanese men and women. J Epidemiol Community Health. 2011;65(3):230–240.

14. Bøhn SK, Ward NC, Hodgson JM, et al. Effects of tea and coffee on cardiovascular disease risk. Food Funct. 2012;3(6):575–591.

83. TEA: GREEN

Introduction

Tea is a widely consumed beverage around the world.[1] Conventional tea is brown or black, a brew of oxidized leaves from the evergreen plant, *Camellia sinensis*.[2] Tea originated in China and spread to the UK, and from there, to the rest of the world. Today, the largest producers of tea in the world are China, India, Kenya and Sri Lanka. Tea was used in early China as a medicinal beverage.[3] Because tea is rich in beneficial polyphenolic compounds, it has garnered considerable medical attention.[4] More recently, several epidemiological and scientific studies have demonstrated that tea consumption has an inverse relationship with cardiovascular diseases.[5] Tea has abundant beneficial bioactive compounds that exhibit anti-inflammatory, anti-oxidative, anti-platelet, anti-vasoconstriction and anti-proliferative effects. They help attenuate cardiovascular risk factors and reduce cardiovascular events, including cardiovascular mortality. Green tea is non-oxidized and constitutes about 20% of the total tea consumed in the world. Green tea may be more cardio-protective than black tea.

Scientific Evidence

- The health beneficial bio-active ingredients in tea are polyphenols. The major polyphenols are catechins and flavonols. Catechins constitute about 80–90% and flavanols about 10% of the total flavonoids in green tea. Catechins include epigallocatechin, epicatechin gallate, and epigallocatechin gallate and epicatechin. Epigallocatechin represents 50 -75% of the total amount of catechins and is the most powerful bioactive polyphenol found in green tea. These compounds have strong anti-oxidant, anti-inflammatory, anti-platelet, anti-vasoconstriction and anti-proliferative effects. These actions help prevent cardiovascular disease.[6]

- Low-density lipoprotein cholesterol oxidation is critical for the development of atherosclerosis, and its prevention helps retard atherosclerosis.[7] Tea and its extracts inhibit low-density lipoprotein cholesterol oxidation.

- Inflammation also plays an important role in atherogenesis. Tea has anti-inflammatory effects.[8]

- Platelet aggregation is intricately involved with acute ischemic cardiac episodes. Tea reduces platelet activation.[9]

- Abnormalities of endothelial function, mainly controlled by nitric oxide, also plays a role in atherogenesis.[10] consumption reverses this endothelial dysfunction and reduces arterial stiffness.

- Epidemiological studies suggest that 1 cup/day of green tea is associated with a 10% decrease in the risk of developing coronary artery disease. In a prospective cohort study, drinking only 2 cups/day of green tea attained a significant reduction in cardiovascular mortality.[11]

- Green tea intake may also help reduce strokes.[12]

Conclusion

Tea, and especially green tea, has a host of bioactive compounds that have beneficial effects on the heart. These beneficial changes help attenuate cardiovascular risk factors, cardiovascular diseases and cardiovascular mortality. Drinking only 2 cups/day of green tea have been shown to exert significant beneficial cardiovascular effects.

Lifestyle Implications

Green tea is more cardioprotective that brown/black tea.

References

1. Weisburger JH. Tea and health: a historical perspective. Cancer Lett. 1997;114(1–2):315–317.
2. Martin, Laura C. (2007). Tea: The Drink that Changed the World. Tuttle Publishing. ISBN 0-8048-3724-4.
3. Chacko SM, Thambi PT, Kuttan R, Nishigaki I. Beneficial effects of green tea: A literature review. Chinese Medicine. 2010;5:13.
4. Balentine DA, Wiseman SA, Bouwens LC. The chemistry of tea flavonoids. Crit Rev Food Sci Nutr. 1997;37 (8):693–704.
5. De Koning Gans JM, Uiterwaal CS, van der Schouw YT, Boer JM, Grobbee DE, Verschuren WM, et al. Tea and coffee consumption and cardiovascular morbidity and mortality. Arterioscler Thromb Vasc Biol. 2010;30:1665–71.
6. Basu A, Lucas EA. Mechanisms and effects of green tea on cardiovascular health. Nutr Rev. 2007 Aug;65(8 Pt 1):361-75.
7. Stocker R, Keaney JF., Jr. The role of oxidative modifications in atherosclerosis. Physiol Rev. 2004;84:1381–478.

8. Neyestani TR, Shariatzade N, Kalayi A, et al. Regular daily intake of black tea improves oxidative stress biomarkers and decreases serum C-reactive protein levels in type 2 diabetic patients. Ann Nutr Metab. 2010;57:40–9.

9. Steptoe A, Gibson EL, Vuononvirta R, Hamer M, Wardle J, Rycroft JA, et al. The effects of chronic tea intake on platelet activation and inflammation: a double-blind placebo controlled trial. Atherosclerosis. 2007;193:277–82.

10. Tabit CE, Chung WB, Hamburg NM, Vita JA. Endothelial dysfunction in diabetes mellitus: molecular mechanisms and clinical implications. Rev Endocr Metab Disord. 2010;11:61–74.

11. Mineharu Y, Koizumi A, Wada Y, et al. Coffee, green tea, black tea and Oolong tea consumption and risk of mortality from cardiovascular disease in Japanese men and women. J Epidemiol Community Health. 2011;65(3):230–240.

12. Wen W, Xiang Y-B, Zheng W, et al. The association of alcohol, tea, and other modifiable lifestyle factors with myocardial infarction and stroke in Chinese men. CVD prevention and control. 2008;3(3):133-140.

84. TURMERIC

Introduction

Turmeric (*Curcuma longa*) plants are members of the ginger family (Zingiberaceae). The rhizome of Curcuma longa, a perennial herb, is boiled, cleaned, and dried, yielding a yellow powder called turmeric. Curcumin, (diferuloylmethane) which gives the yellow color to turmeric, is a major component of turmeric and is commonly used as a spice or a food-coloring agent. Its essential oils are also used in perfumes. Commercially, it is used as a dye for textiles and culturally, as a pigment for skin in ceremonial functions. Its medicinal use goes back several centuries, especially in Ayurveda. Curcumin has been shown to exhibit antioxidant, anti-inflammatory,[1] antiviral, antibacterial, antifungal, antiamyloid and anticancer activitie.[2] Its use has therefore been investigated in a wide variety of diseases.[3] Its anti-inflammatory and anti-oxidant effects have ignited a healthy therapeutic curiosity regarding its beneficial effects in cardiovascular diseases.[4] It also has favorable effects on the lipid profile.[5]

Scientific Evidence

- Curcumin, 500 mg orally once a day decreased lipid peroxides by 44%, total serum cholesterol by 11.63%, and increased serum high density lipoprotein cholesterol levels by 29%, in healthy volunteers.[5]

- In patients with acute coronary syndrome, low doses of curcumin taken 15 mg, three times daily for 2 months, resulted in reductions in total and low-density lipoprotein cholesterol levels and elevations in high-density lipoprotein cholesterol levels.[6]

- In animal studies, oral administration of turmeric extract inhibits low density lipoprotein cholesterol oxidation. This beneficial antioxidant effect has also been noted in human subjects.[7]

- There have been reductions in body mass index and glycated hemoglobin (HbAic) noted with curcumin in diabetics. Curcumin protects the function of β-cells, and helps prevent pre-diabetics from progressing to overt diabetes.[8]

- Curcumin has significant anti-inflammatory actions that are cardioprotective.[3]

- Endothelial function improvement has been noted in animal studies as well as humans with the ingestion of this spice,[9] including protection against Adriamycin (an anti-cancer drug) induced cardiomyopathy.[10]

Conclusion

Turmeric is high in curcumin, a polyphenol. This agent has significant health benefits — especially, its ingestion may help in the prevention of cardiovascular disorders. It has anti-lipid, anti-inflammatory and anti-oxidant actions which help attenuate several processes involved in the pathophysiology of cardiovascular disease.

Lifestyle Implications

Dietary supplementation with curcumin is beneficial for cardiovascular health. The curcumin rich spice turmeric, prominently used in Indian cooking, should be in every kitchen.

References

1. Menon VP, Sudheer AR. Antioxidant and anti-inflammatory properties of curcumin. Adv Exp Med Biol. 2007;595:105-25.
2. Zhou H, Beevers CS, Huang S. The targets of curcumin. Curr Drug Targets. 2011 Mar 1;12(3):332-47.
3. Aggarwal BB, Harikumar KB. Potential therapeutic effects of curcumin, the anti-inflammatory agent, against neurodegenerative, cardiovascular, pulmonary, metabolic, autoimmune and neoplastic diseases. Int J Biochem Cell Biol. 2009 Jan;41(1):40-59.
4. Kapakos G, Youreva V, Srivastava AK. Cardiovascular protection by curcumin: molecular aspects. Indian J Biochem Biophys. 2012 Oct;49(5):306-15.
5. Soni K.B., Kuttan R. Effect of oral curcumin administration on serum peroxides and cholesterol levels in human volunteers. Indian J. Physiol. Pharmacol. 1992;36:273–275.
6. Alwi I., Santoso T., Suyono S., Sutrisna B., Suyatna F.D., Kresno S.B., Ernie S. The effect of curcumin on lipid level in patients with acute coronary syndrome. Acta Med. Indones. 2008;40:201–210.
7. Ramirez-Bosca A, Soler A, Carrion MA, et al. An hydroalcoholic extract of curcuma longa lowers the apo B/apo A ratio. Implications for atherogenesis prevention. Mechanisms of ageing and development. 2000;119:41-7.

8. Chuengsamarn S, Rattanamongkolgul S, Luechapudiporn R, Phisalaphong C, Jirawatnotai S. Curcumin Extract for Prevention of Type 2 Diabetes. Diabetes Care. 2012;35(11):2121-2127.

9. Akazawa N., Choi Y., Miyaki A., Tanabe Y., Sugawara J., Ajisaka R., Maeda S. Curcumin ingestion and exercise training improve vascular endothelial function in postmenopausal women. Nutr. Res. 2012;32:795–799.

10. Mohamad RH, El-Bastawesy AM, Zekry ZK, et al. The role of Curcuma longa against doxorubicin (adriamycin)-induced toxicity in rats. J Med Food. 2009 Apr;12(2):394-402.

85. VACATION

Introduction

According to Wikepedia, "a vacation or holiday is a leave of absence from a regular occupation or a specific trip or journey, usually for the purpose of recreation or tourism". Vacationing, like other recreational activities such as hobbies, socializing etc have been associated with a littany of well-being outcomes. These include psychological well-being,[1,2] and an improved physical status.[3,4] Vacations lead to less severe disease outcomes,[5] and increased longevity.[6,7] Cardiovascular benefits have also been noted in vacationers.

Scientific Evidence

- In a study of middle aged men at risk of developing coronary heart disease, taking vacations resulted in several health benefits: a 17% reduction in all-cause mortality, a 29% reduction in cardiovascular mortality, and a 32% reduction in coronary heart disease and heart attacks.[8,9]
- In a 20-year study, researchers found that women who took vacation once every six years or less were almost eight times more likely to develop coronary heart disease or have a heart attack than women who took at least two vacations per year.[10]
- A study from the Mind Body Center at the University of Pittsburgh, surveyed 1,399 participants recruited for studies on cardiovascular disease, breast cancer and other conditions. Researchers found that leisure activities, including taking vacations, contributed to higher positive emotional levels and less depression among the participants. In another study, participants felt greater vitality and decreased distress after a week of vacation at a resort, with the benefits on depression lasting even during the tenth month post vacation.[11]

Conclusion

A journey outside often reaps benefits inside. Substantial scientific data supports the psychological and physical benefits of vacations. The cardiovascular benefits have also been well documented.

Lifestyle Implications

Vacations are good for your health — and the cardiovascular system.

References

1. Diener E, Lucas RE, Oishi S. Subjective well-being: the science of happiness and life satisfaction. In: Snyder CR, Lopez SJ, editors. Handbook of Positive Psychology. New York: Oxford University Press; 2002.
2. Ryff CD, Singer BH, Dienberg Love G. Positive health: connecting well-being with biology. Philos Trans R Soc Lond B Biol Sci. 2004;359:1383–94.
3. Ulrich RS, Simons RF, Losito BD, Fiorito E, Miles MA, Zelson M. Stress recovery during exposure to natural and urban environments. J Environ Psychol. 1991;11:201–30.
4. Staats H, Gatersleben B, Hartig T. Change in mood as a function of environmental design: arousal and pleasure on a simulated forest hike. J Environ Psychol. 1997;17:283–300.
5. Cohen S, Doyle WJ, Skoner DP, Rabin BS, Gwaltney JM., Jr Social ties and susceptibility to the common cold. JAMA. 1997;277:1940–4.
6. Gump BB, Matthews KA. Are vacations good for your health? The 9-year mortality experience after the multiple risk factor intervention trial. Psychosom Med. 2000;62:608–12.
7. Tominaga K, Andow J, Koyama Y, Numao S, Kurokawa E, Ojima M, Nagai M. Family environment, hobbies and habits as psychosocial predictors of survival for surgically treated patients with breast cancer. Jpn J Clin Oncol. 1998;28:36–4122–24.
8. Multiple Risk Factor Intervention Trial Risk Factor Changes and Mortality Results. JAMA. 1982;248(12):1465–1477.
9. Gump BB, Matthews KA. Are vacations good for your health? The 9-year mortality experience after the multiple risk factor intervention trial. Psychosom Med. 2000 Sep-Oct;62(5):608-12.
10. Elaine D. Eaker, Joan Pinsky, William P. Castelli; Myocardial Infarction and Coronary Death among Women: Psychosocial Predictors from a 20-Year Follow-up of Women in the Framingham Study, American Journal of Epidemiology, Volume 135, Issue 8, 15 April 1992, Pages 854–864.
11. Epel ES, Puterman E, Lin J, et al. Meditation and vacation effects have an impact on disease-associated molecular phenotypes. Translational Psychiatry. 2016;6(8): e880.

86. VACCINATION

Introduction

Vaccination against influenza was recommended for the 2016-2017 season by the Advisory Committee on Immunization Practices for everyone 6 months and older with either the inactivated influenza vaccine or the recombinant influenza vaccine.[1] Influenza remains a serious disease in the USA and can lead to hospitalization and sometimes even death. Influenza vaccine is recommended every year due to declining antibodies over time and the constantly changing nature of the flu virus. The vaccination reduces hospitalization and deaths from influenza. It also reduces cardiovascular mortality.[2] Increasing evidence is also highlighting the cardiovascular protective benefits of pneumococcal pneumonia vaccination.[3]

Scientific Evidence

- During influenza epidemics, hospitalizations for cerebrovascular and cardiovascular diseases increase.[4] Acute infections, common in those not vaccinated, such as upper respiratory tract infections, also tend to increase the risk of cardiovascular,[5] and cerebrovascular events.[6]

- Several small observational studies have suggested that influenza vaccination may be associated with a reduction in the risk of cardiac arrest,[7] myocardial infarction,[8] and acute cerebrovascular events.[9]

- In a small, unblinded, controlled trial, vaccination was also associated with lower rates of death, myocardial infarction, or revascularization among persons with acute coronary syndromes and those scheduled to undergo percutaneous coronary intervention.[10]

- Pneumococcal vaccination is also helpful in preventing hospitalization and cardiovascular events.[11] In a meta-analytic review of eleven studies involving 332,267 subjects, researchers concluded that pneumococcal vaccination was associated with a decreased risk of cardiovascular events and mortality.[12]

Conclusion

There is robust evidence based data that influenza and pneumococcal vaccination prevents major cardiovascular events, especially in the elderly. According to the Centers for Disease Control and Prevention, "all persons aged 6 months or older who do not have a contraindication should receive annual influenza vaccination with an age-appropriate formulation of inactivated influenza vaccine (IIV) or recombinant influenza vaccine (RIV). Adults who are immunocompetent and aged 65 years or older should receive 13-valent pneumococcal conjugate vaccine (PCV13) followed by 23-valent pneumococcal polysaccharide vaccine (PPSV23) at least 1 year after PCV13." These vaccinations provide some protection against cardiovascular events. Your physician will be able to advise you on which vaccination to take and when, depending on your age and health.

Lifestyle Implications

Get vaccinated as recommended by the Centers for Disease Control and Prevention. Both influenza and pneumococcal vaccination reduce cardiovascular events, including mortality.

References

1. https://www.cdc.gov/flu/protect/keyfacts.htm (Accessed May 5, 2017)
2. Kristin L. Nichol, James Nordin, John Mullooly, et al. Influenza Vaccination and Reduction in Hospitalizations for Cardiac Disease and Stroke among the Elderly. N Engl J Med 2003; 348:1322-1332.
3. Vila-Corcoles A, Ochoa-Gondar O, Rodriguez-Blanco T, et al. Clinical effectiveness of pneumococcal vaccination against acute myocardial infarction and stroke in people over 60 years: the CAPAMIS study, one-year follow-up. BMC Public Health. 2012 Mar 22;12:222.
4. Bainton D, Jones GR, Hole D. Influenza and ischemic heart disease -- a possible trigger for acute myocardial infarction? Int J Epidemiol 1978;7:231-239.
5. Meier CR, Jick SS, Derby LE, Vasilakis C, Jick H. Acute respiratory-tract infections and risk of first-time acute myocardial infarction. Lancet 1998;351:1467-1471.
6. Becher H, Grau A, Steindorf K, Buggle F, Hacke W. Previous infection and other risk factors for acute cerebrovascular ischaemia: attributable risks and the characterisation of high risk groups. J Epidemiol Biostat 2000;5:277-283.
7. Siscovick DS, Raghunathan RE, Lin D, et al. Influenza vaccination and the risk of primary cardiac arrest. Am J Epidemiol 2000;152:674-677.

8.   Naghavi M, Barlas Z, Siadaty S, et al. Association of influenza vaccination and reduced risk of recurrent myocardial infarction. Circulation 2000;102:3039-3045.

9.   Lavallee P, Perchaud V, Gautier-Bertrand M, Grabli D, Amarenco P. Association between influenza vaccination and reduced risk of brain infarction. Stroke 2002;33:513-518 ([Erratum, Stroke 2002;33:1171).

10.   Gurfinkel EP, de la Fuente L, Mendiz O, Mautner B. Influenza vaccine pilot study in acute coronary syndromes and planned percutaneous coronary interventions: the FLU Vaccination Acute Coronary Syndromes (FLUVACS) Study. Circulation 2002;105:2143-2147.

11.   Hung IF, Leung AY, Chu DW, et al. Prevention of acute myocardial infarction and stroke among elderly persons by dual pneumococcal and influenza vaccination: a prospective cohort study. Clin Infect Dis. 2010;51:1007-16.

12.   Vlachopoulos CV, Terentes-Printzios DG, Aznaouridis KA, Pietri PG, Stefanadis C. Association between pneumococcal vaccination and cardiovascular outcomes: a systematic review and meta-analysis of cohort studies. Eur J Prev Cardiol. 2015 Sep;22(9):1185-99.

87. VEGETABLES

Introduction

A high daily intake of plant based foods promotes health. Although fruits
and vegetable are usually lumped together, when it comes to health benefits,
a distinction may exist between their intake, composition and benefits.[1]
Besides providing energy, vegetables are rich in a number of bioactive
compounds, including vitamins, minerals, antioxidants, carotenoids and
flavonoids. They are also high in fiber. Bioactive ingredients vary from
vegetable to vegetable. For example, unskinned potatoes are rich in starch,
protein, vitamin C, and potassium and also provide dietary fiber. Tomatoes
on the other hand are rich in lycopene, while carrots are rich in carotenoids.
Increasing scientific evidence indicates that eating more vegetables protects
against many chronic diseases, including type 2 diabetes, dementia,
depression and some cancers. There is also a reduction in all-cause
mortality.[2] The role of vegetable consumption in decreasing the risk of
hypertension, coronary heart disease and stroke is also well documented.
There is a reduction in cardiovascular mortality.

Scientific Evidence

- The Dietary Approaches to Stop Hypertension style diet results in
  a lower blood pressure. This diet is rich in fruits and vegetables.[3]
- A systematic review and meta-analysis of six studies showed that a
  greater intake of green leafy vegetables was associated with a 14%
  reduction in risk of type 2 diabetes.[4]
- He and associates studied data from eight studies. These included
  257,551 individuals (sustaining 4917 stroke events) for an average
  follow-up of 13 years. Compared with individuals who had less
  than three servings of fruit and vegetables per day to those with
  consumption of more than five servings per day, the latter group
  had a reduced risk of stroke.[5]
- In a prospective population-based cohort study, 20,069 men and
  women aged 20 to 65 years, free of cardiovascular disease, agreed
  to be monitored via a 178-item habitual food consumption
  questionnaire. This study found that those with a higher vegetable
  intake had reduced coronary heart disease.[6]

- He and his collegues observed that participants consuming more than 391 g/day of fruit and vegetables had a 17% lower risk of non-fatal and fatal coronary heart disease incidence than those who consumed less than 235 g/day.[7]
- There is also a reduction in cardiovascular mortality with increased vegetable consumption.[8]

Conclusion

Several major reviews have shown the powerful disease prevention potential associated with an increase in consumption of vegetables. Vegetarian diets have been promoted since the 18th century by humans in search of a better physical and spiritual health.[9] Evidence based data now supports the health benefits accrued from eating a plant based diet.

Lifestyle Implications

Eat more vegetables — the more colorful your choice, the better the health benefit.

References

1. Appleton KM, Hemingway A, Saulais L, et al. Increasing vegetable intakes: rationale and systematic review of published interventions. European Journal of Nutrition. 2016;55:869-896.
2. Leenders M, Sluijs I, Ros MM, Boshuizen HC, et al. Fruit and vegetable consumption and mortality: European prospective investigation into cancer and nutrition. Am J Epidemiol. 2013 Aug 15;178(4):590-602.
3. Appel LJ, Moore TJ, Obarzanek E, Vollmer WM, Svetkey LP, Sacks FM, Bray GA, Vogt TM, Cutler JA, Windhauser MM, et al. A clinical trial of the effects of dietary patterns on blood pressure. DASH Collaborative Research Group. N Engl J Med. 1997;336:1117–24.
4. Carter P, Gray LJ, Troughton J, Khunti K, Davies MJ. Fruit and vegetable intake and incidence of type 2 diabetes mellitus: systematic review and meta-analysis. BMJ. 2010;341:c4229.
5. He FJ, Nowson CA, MacGregor GA. Fruit and vegetable consumption and stroke: meta-analysis of cohort studies. Lancet. 2006;367:320–326.
6. Oude Griep LM, Geleijnse JM, Kromhout D, Ocké MC, Verschuren WMM. Raw and Processed Fruit and Vegetable Consumption and 10-Year Coronary Heart Disease Incidence in a Population-Based Cohort Study in the Netherlands. Tomé D, ed. PLoS ONE. 2010;5(10): e13609.
7. He FJ, Nowson CA, Lucas M, MacGregor GA. Increased consumption of fruit and vegetables is related to a reduced risk of coronary heart disease: meta-analysis of cohort studies. J Hum Hypertens. 2007;21:717–728.

8. Wang X, Ouyang Y, Liu J, Zhu M, Zhao G, Bao W, et al. Fruit and vegetable consumption and mortality from all causes, cardiovascular disease, and cancer: systematic review and dose–response meta-analysis of prospective cohort studies. BMJ. 2014;349: g4490.

9. Roe DA. History of promotion of vegetable cereal diets. J Nutr. 1986;116:1355–63.

88. VINEGAR

Introduction

Vinegar originated from the French 'vin aigre', and means "sour wine". It has a long history. According to Johnston and Gass,[1] vinegar was discovered in Babylonia (c. 5000 BC) and used as a food preservative. Vinegar has also been used for medicinal purposes during ancient times. Hippocrates (c. 420 BC) used it to manage wounds, while Sung Tse, the 10th century creator of forensic medicine, used sulfur and vinegar to wash hands to avoid infection during autopsies. Made from fermenting carbohydrates, usually fruits and grains, alcohol is first formed by yeasts. The acetic acid bacteria (Acetobacter) then convert this alcohol to acetic acid. Commercially available vinegar usually contains about 5–20% acetic acid and is commonly used in cooking, in pickling or as a salad dressing.

Scientific Evidence

- Major studies in humans on the beneficial effects of vinegar in attenuating the incidence, severity and complications of cardiovascular diseases are lacking. However, several studies, both in animals and humans, suggest that regular vinegar ingestion may be beneficial for the cardiovascular health.[2]
- Vinegar reduces blood pressure in rats,[3] probably via inhibiting the renin-angiotensin hormonal system.[4]
3. Vinegar has beneficial effects on body weight and triglyceride levels.[5]
4. Vinegar exhibits an anti-glycemic effect, both in healthy,[6] and diabetic subjects.[7]
5. People with vinegar consumption exhibit higher antioxidant activity.[8]
6. Vinegar inhibits platelet aggregation,[9] has antithrombotic effects,[10] and improves blood fluidity.[11]

Conclusion

Vinegar demonstrates cardiovascular friendly actions. However, robust human studies elucidating the vinegar related cardiovascular benefits remain lacking. The non-professional literature states that apple cider vinegar is the most popular consumed vinegar by the general public. If you like vinegar as a salad dressing, continue using it or you could drink apple cider vinegar in an amount of 2 tsp. in water or juice daily.

Lifestyle Implications

Regular ingestion of vinegar, for example as a salad dressing, may have cardioprotective effects.

References

1. Carol S. Johnston, Cindy A. Gaas. Vinegar: Medicinal Uses and Antiglycemic Effect. MedGenMed. 2006; 8(2): 61-63.
2. P Mitrou, E Petsiou, E Papakonstantinou, et al. The role of acetic acid on glucose uptake and blood flow rates in the skeletal muscle in humans with impaired glucose tolerance. European Journal of Clinical Nutrition (2015) 69, 734–739.
3. Kondo S, Tayama K, Tsukamoto Y, Ikeda K, Yamori Y. Antihypertensive effects of acetic acid and vinegar on spontaneously hypertensive rats. Biosci Biotechnol Biochem. 2001;65:2690–2694.31.
4. Honsho S, Sugiyama A, Takahara A, Satoh Y, Nakamura Y, Hashimoto K. A red wine vinegar beverage can inhibit the renninangiotensin system: experimental evidence in vivo. Biol Pharm Bull. 2005;28:1208–1211.
5. Tomoo Kondo, Mikiya Kishi, Takashi Fushimi, Shinobu Ugajin, and Takayuki Kaga. Vinegar Intake Reduces Body Weight, Body Fat Mass, and Serum Triglyceride Levels in Obese Japanese Subjects. Bioscience, Biotechnology, And Biochemistry Vol. 73, Iss. 8, 2009.
6. Johnston CS, Steplewska I, Long CA, Harris LN, Ryals RH. Examination of the antiglycemic properties of vinegar in healthy adults. Ann Nutr Metab 2010; 56: 74-79.
7. Johnston CS, Kim CM, Buller AJ. Vinegar improves insulin sensitivity to a highcarbohydrate meal in subjects with insulin resistance or type 2 diabetes. Diabetes. Care 2004; 27: 281–282.
8. Xu, Q.P, Tao, W.Y, Ao, Z.H, 2007. Antioxidant activity of vinegar melanoidins. Food Chem. 102, 841–849.
9. Jing Li, Guoyong Yu, Junfeng Fan. Alditols and monosaccharides from sorghum vinegar can attenuate platelet aggregation by inhibiting cyclooxygenase-1 and thromboxane-A2 synthase. Journal of Ethnopharmacology 155 (2014) 285–292.
10. He, L.W, Li, Z.M, Sun, Y, Zhang, Y.Y, Fan, J.F, 2012. Effect of acetic acid and low molecular weight component of mature vinegar on platelet aggregation. Food Nutr. China 18 (8), 65–67.
11. Yamagishi, K., Kimura, T., Kameyama, M., Nagata, T., et al., 1998. Purification and identification of blood fluidity improvement factor in brewed rice vinegar (Kurosu). J. Jpn. Soc. Food Sci. 45, 545–549.

89. VITAMIN D

Introduction

Vitamin D, also called calciferol, exists as Vitamin D2 (ergocalciferol), which is largely ingested and Vitamin D3 (cholecalciferol), which is synthesized in human body. Because the majority of vitamin D is synthetized in the human epidermis via ultraviolet irradiation, it is often called the "sunshine vitamin". Sunlight related sythesis in the human epidermis is responsible for almost 80% of the human vitamin D supply. Vitamin D levels should be >30 ng/mL, and vitamin D intoxication is considered if these exceed >150 ng/mL.[1] Its deficiency has been associated with increased risk for many chronic diseases including autoimmune diseases, some cancers, infectious disease, schizophrenia and type 2 diabetes[2] Low vitamin D levels may also increase cardiovascular risk.[3] Deficiency has been noted in various cardiovascular conditions such atherosclerosis, coronary artery disease and stroke.

Scientific Evidence

- Some studies have suggested that vitamin D deficiency is associated with higher blood pressure levels, while others find this association not consistent.[4] A connection of low vitamin D levels with obesity,[5] and lower high-density lipoprotein cholesterol and higher triglycerides, as well as higher apolipoprotein E levels, has also been noted.[6] Some studies have failed to establish this relationship.

- A meta-analysis of 11 prospective studies involving 3,612 cases and 55,713 noncase participants provided evidence for a strong inverse association between vitamin D levels and incidence of type 2 diabetes.[7] A similar association has also been noted with peripheral artery disease.

- In a study of 1,739 participants from the Framingham Offspring cohort, researchers found that a vitamin D concentration below 15 ng/mL was consistently associated with an increased risk of cardiovascular events. They estimated that patients with vitamin D deficiency had a 5-year rate of developing a cardiovascular event two times higher than in those with adequate vitamin D stores.[8] A clear association between vitamin D status and the occurrence of acute myocardial infarction and coronary heart disease has however not been firmly established.

- In a meta-analysis of seven studies, involving 47,809 individuals and 926 cerebrovascular events, the risk for cerebrovascular disease was significantly lower in subjects with high 25(OH)D levels compared to those with low levels.[9]
- Low vitamin D levels are also associated with an increase in cardiovascular mortality and overall mortality. Claims that vitamin D supplementation decreases mortality have been unconvincing.[10]
- Low vitamin D levels result in vascular inflammation, decreased insulin sensitivity, endothelial dysfunction, formation of foam cells, and proliferation of smooth muscle cells – changes that favor atherosclerosis.

Conclusion

Adequate Vitamin D levels should help in preventing, reducing the severity, and enhancing improvement of several chronic diseases. For a light skinned person, 10 to 15 minutes of sun exposure followed by good sun protection should be sufficient to produce adequate vitamin D. Vitamin D2 or D3 can also be taken up via nutrition, where it is present in small amounts – for example in eggs, mushrooms and fish.

Lifestyle Implications

Get adequate sun exposure daily. Vitamin D is synthesized in the skin and adequate levels appear to be important for good cardiovascular health.

References

1. Holick M. F., Chen T. C. Vitamin D deficiency: a worldwide problem with health consequences. The American Journal of Clinical Nutrition. 2008;87(4, supplement):1080S–1086S.
2. Wacker M, Holick MF. Sunlight and Vitamin D: A global perspective for health. Dermato-endocrinology. 2013;5(1):51-108.
3. Kienreich K., Tomaschitz A., Verheyen N., et al. Vitamin D and cardiovascular disease. Nutrients. 2013;5(8):3005–3021.
4. Witham M.D., Nadir M.A., Struthers A.D. Effect of vitamin D on blood pressure: A systematic review and meta-analysis. J. Hypertens. 2009;27:1948–1954.
5. Earthman C.P., Beckman L.M., Masodkar K., Sibley S.D. The link between obesity and low 25-hydroxyvitamin D concentrations: Considerations and implications. Int. J. Obes. (Lond.) 2012;36:387–396.

6. Jorde R., Grimnes G. Vitamin D and metabolic health with special reference to the effect of vitamin D on serum lipids. Prog. Lipid Res. 2011;50:303–312.

7. Forouhi NG, Ye Z, Rickard AP, et al. Circulating 25-hydroxyvitamin D concentration and the risk of type 2 diabetes: results from the European Prospective Investigation into Cancer (EPIC)-Norfolk cohort and updated meta-analysis of prospective studies. Diabetologia. 2012;55(8):2173–2182.

8. Wang TJ, Pencina MJ, Booth SL, et al. Vitamin D deficiency and risk of cardiovascular disease. Circulation. 2008;117(4):503–511.

9. Chowdhury R., Stevens S., Ward H., Chowdhury S., Sajjad A., Franco O.H. Circulating vitamin D, calcium and risk of cerebrovascular disease: A systematic review and meta-analysis. Eur. J. Epidemiol. 2012;27:581–591.

10. Zittermann A., Prokop S. The role of vitamin D for cardiovascular disease and overall mortality. Advances in Experimental Medicine and Biology. 2014;810:106–119.

90. VITAMINS: MULTIVITAMINS

Introduction

A vitamin is an organic compound that is needed in small amounts for the normal growth and proper working of the human body. Vitamins may be grouped as fat soluble (A, D, E, and K) or water soluble (vitamins B and C). A multivitamin preparation may contain several vitamins and minerals such as potassium, iodine, selenium, borate, zinc, calcium, magnesium, manganese, molybdenum, betacarotene, and iron. Many US adults take vitamin supplements,[1] to prevent chronic diseases,[2] or for a good general health and well-being.[3] However, most published data suggests that indiscriminate consumption of multivitamins may be associated with worse health outcomes, including premature mortality.

Scientific Evidence

- Supplementation with beta carotene, vitamin A, and vitamin E may increase mortality. In a review of 47 studies involving 181,000 participants, researchers reported that taking vitamin A supplements increased the risk of death by 16%, beta-carotene by 7%, and vitamin E by 4%.[4]
- A large study of 38,772 older women, enrolled in the Iowa Women's Health Study, revealed that dietary vitamin and mineral supplements were associated with an increased total mortality risk.[5]
- In another large study of 14,641 male US physicians, aged 50 years or older, a daily multivitamin intake was not associated with any reduction in major cardiovascular events such as myocardial infarction, stroke, or cardiovascular mortality, after more than a decade of treatment and follow-up.[6]
- Some studies have even indicated a worse health outcome in certain diseases with the use of multivitamins. High levels of multivitamin intake along with other supplements may increase the risk of advanced and fatal prostate.[7]

Conclusion

Vitamins supplementation is not cardioprotective. Scientific evidence does not support their use in reducing cardiovascular events, including cardiovascular mortality. Evidence based data even suggests that multivitamin usage may result in an increase in mortality. Individual vitamins or multivitamins should only be taken if prescribed by a health care provider for specific deficiencies or conditions.

Lifestyle Implications

For cardiovascular protection, skip multivitamins. Instead, invest in a balanced, nutritious diet, high in whole grains, fruits and vegetables, and low in calories, saturated fat, trans fat and sodium.

References

1. Timbo BB, Ross MP, McCarthy PV, Lin CT. Dietary supplements in a national survey: prevalence of use and reports of adverse events. J Am Diet Assoc. 2006;106(12):1966-1974.
2. Ervin RB, Wright JD, Kennedy-Stephenson J. Use of dietary supplements in the United States, 1988-94. Vital Health Stat 11. 1999;11(244): i-iii, 1-14
3. Blendon RJ, DesRoches CM, Benson JM, Brodie M, Altman DE. Americans' views on the use and regulation of dietary supplements. Arch Intern Med. 2001;161(6):805-810.
4. Bjelakovic G, Nikolova D, Gluud LL, Simonetti RG, Gluud C. Mortality in randomized trials of antioxidant supplements for primary and secondary prevention: systematic review and meta-analysis. JAMA. 2007 Feb 28;297(8):842-57.
5. Mursu J, Robien K, Harnack LJ, Park K, Jacobs DR Jr. Dietary supplements and mortality rate in older women: the Iowa Women's Health Study. Arch Intern Med. 2011 Oct 10;171(18):1625-33.
6. Sesso HD, Christen WG, Bubes V, Smith JP, MacFadyen J, Schvartz M, Manson JE, Glynn RJ, Buring JE, Gaziano JM. Multivitamins in the Prevention of Cardiovascular Disease in MenThe Physicians' Health Study II Randomized Controlled Trial. JAMA. 2012;308(17):1751–1760.
7. Lawson KA, Wright ME, Subar A, Mouw T, et al, Multivitamin use and risk of prostate cancer in the National Institutes of Health-AARP Diet and Health Study. J Natl Cancer Inst. 2007 May 16;99(10):754-64.

91. WAIST SIZE

Introduction

The waist is the part between the ribs and the hips – and waist size measurements can provide information regarding the risk for cardiovascular disease. Typically, the smallest waist size is measured, usually just above the belly button for women and just below the belly button for men. According to the National Heart, Lung, and Blood Institute, men who have a waist circumference greater than 40 inches (102 cm) and women who have a waist circumference greater than 35 inches (88 cm) are at higher risk of cardiovascular diseases.[1] Waist–hip ratio is the ratio of the circumference of the waist to that of the hips. Waist–hip ratios of 0.7 for women and 0.9 for men have been shown to correlate strongly with good general health. According to the World Health Organization, a waist–hip ratio above 0.85 in females and above 0.9 is males is indicative of obesity. If the fat is distributed mainly around the waist, the body is often described as "apple-shaped" (these people have high amounts of visceral abdominal fat) and these people suffer from greater health risks than those with a "pear-shaped" body, which carries more weight around the hips.[2] A person's waist-to-height ratio (WHtR), is defined as their waist circumference divided by their height, both being measured in the same units. WHtR is also a measure of the distribution of body fat. Higher values correlate with increased visceral abdominal fat stores and prognosticate a higher risk of obesity-related cardiovascular diseases.[3] These three anthrometric measurements help identify people with excess visceral fat. High amounts of visceral fat is strongly related to a clustering of cardiovascular risk factors and increased incidence of cardiovascular diseases and premature death.[4] Body mass index, although commonly used as a measurement to define obesity, does not take into account the distribution of fat around the body.[5]

Scientific Evidence

- Higher waist circumference correlates with a higher degree of visceral adiposity and is associated with higher levels of blood pressure, insulin, triglycerides, total cholesterol, and diabetes, and lower levels of high-density lipoprotein cholesterol.[6]

- Higher waist circumference is associated with a higher all-cause mortality. In a pooled analysis of 11 cohort studies with over 650,000 adults.[7] In this study, men experienced a reduction of 3 years and women a reduction of 5 years in life expectancy, when those with the highest versus lowest waist circumference were compared. Higher waist circumference was also associated with an increase in cardiovascular deaths.

- Abnormal waist-hip ratio is associated with increased visceral fat and is associated with an increased risk for abnormal lipid levels, hypertension and type 2 diabetes, in both men and women. It also correlates with premature death. An association has also been seen with sleep apnea – another risk factor for cardiovascular disease. Pear shaped people have a reduced risk of metabolic complications.

- WHtR measurements may also be a good screening tool for visceral obesity. Patients with abnormal WhtR have a higher degree of atherosclerosis.[8] WHtR may be a better measure of the risk of heart disease, heart attack, stroke and coronary heart disease mortality.

Conclusion

Evidence based data confirms that the three waist measurements mentioned above help identify visceral obesity – increased visceral fat is associated with a higher risk for ischemic heart disease, stroke and premature death.

Lifestyle Implications

Monitor your waist size – it may be a stronger indicator of your cardiovascular risk and premature death risk, than your weight alone.

References

1. http://www.scielosp.org/pdf/rpsp/v10n2/5870.pdf (accessed May 6, 2017).
2. Jensen MD. Role of body fat distribution and the metabolic complications of obesity. J Am Coll Cardiol. 2008;93(11_supplement_1): s57–s63.
3. Browning, L., Hsieh, S., & Ashwell, M. (2010). A systematic review of waist-to-height ratio as a screening tool for the prediction of cardiovascular disease and diabetes: 0·5 could be a suitable global boundary value. Nutrition Research Reviews, 23(2), 247-269.

4. Jensen MD. Health consequences of fat distribution. Horm Res. 1997;48 Suppl 5:88-92.

5. Gopinath S, Ganesh BA, Manoj K, Rubiya. Comparision between body mass index and abdominal obesity for the screening for diabetes in healthy individuals. Indian Journal of Endocrinology and Metabolism. 2012;16 (Suppl 2): S441-S442.

6. Reis JP, Allen N, Gunderson EP, et al. Excess Body Mass Index- and Waist Circumference-Years and Incident Cardiovascular Disease: The CARDIA Study. Obesity (Silver Spring, Md). 2015;23(4):879-885.

7. James R. Cerhan, Steven C. Moore, Eric J. Jacobs, et al. A Pooled Analysis of Waist Circumference and Mortality in 650,000 Adults. Mayo Clin Proc. 2014 March; 89(3): 335–345.

8. Oh HG, Nallamshetty S, Rhee EJ. Increased risk of progression of coronary artery calcification in male subjects with high baseline waist-to-height ratio: the Kangbuk Samsung health study. Diabetes Metab J 2016;40:54–61.

92. WATER

Introduction

Water covers over 70% of the earth. It is the most common liquid on earth. It is a tasteless, colorless and odorless liquid that is essential for human life. Over 50% of the human body is made up of water. Humans do not store water and need to drink about 1.5 liters of water per day.[1] and can survive only a day or two without it. Water serves a host of functions in the human body, including bringing oxygen and nutrients to the cells, helping in several chemical and metabolic reactions in the cells and in the removal of waste products. It is the main component of blood and helps in temperature regulation of the body. Adequate and clean water intake may also play a role in preventing disease and maintaining good cardiovascular health.

Scientific Evidence

- A study showed that intake of natural mineral water, rich in sodium bicarbonate, reduced low-density lipoprotein cholesterol levels and several cardiovascular risk indexes (total-cholesterol/ low-density lipoprotein cholesterol ratio and low-density lipoprotein cholesterol/ high-density lipoprotein cholesterol ratio).[2] Another study showed that intake of sodium rich bicarbonate water helps reduce cardiovascular risks in postmenopausal women.[3]

- Obesity is a major risk factor for cardiovascular disease. Drinking water instead of other beverages, and drinking water in greater volume, is one method practiced in weight management.[4] Water may also positively alter the body metabolism.[5]

- Drinking hard water has been inversely related to cardiovascular diseases.[6] Hard water is richer in calcium and magnesium. Calcium in hard water helps reduce blood pressure.[7]

- Water rich in magnesium (hard water) may also help in preventing cardiac arrhythmias.[8] Drinking water rich in magnesium may thus be cardiovascular protective.

- Water drank at room temperature or colder, when compared to drinking body tempered water, had beneficial cardiovascular effects in the short term, including an increase in the cardiac vagal tone and a corresponding decrease in heart rate and decreased workload of the heart.[9]

- Water contaminated with arsenic is harmful to the cardiovascular health. It accelerates atherosclerosis and increases ischemic heart disease deaths.[10]
- Human drinking water in industrialized cities may contain many pharmaceutically active chemicals, the potential harmful cardiovascular effects of which are unknown.

Conclusion

Water should be imbibed at room temperature or colder. It should ideally be rich in minerals like sodium bicarbonate and magnesium. Hard water is naturally high in calcium and magnesium and may be cardiovascular protective. Water should be free of arsenic and potentially harmful industrial chemical compounds. Excessive or low intake of water can be harmful.

Lifestyle Implications

Drink adequate amounts of water a day. In general, tap water is healthy, although clean natural mineral water appears to be somewhat more beneficial for cardiovascular health.

References

1.	Montain SJ, Latzka WA, Sawka MN. Fluid replacement recommendations for training in hot weather. Mil Med. 1999 Jul;164(7):502-8.
2.	Perez-Granados, A.M.; Navas-Carretero, S.; Schoppen, S., et al. Reduction in cardiovascular risk by sodium-bicarbonated mineral water in moderately hypercholesterolemic young adults. J. Nutr. Biochem. 2010, 21, 948–953.
3.	Schoppen S, Pérez-Granados AM, Carbajal A, et al. A sodium-rich carbonated mineral water reduces cardiovascular risk in postmenopausal women. J Nutr. 2004 May;134(5):1058-63.
4.	Centers for Disease Control and Prevention, Division of Nutrition, Physical Activity and Obesity (CDC) Rethink Your Drink.available online: http://www.cdc.gov/healthyweight/healthy_eating/drinks.html.
5.	Stookey J.D., Constant F., Popkin B.M., Gardner C.D. Drinking water is associated with weight loss in overweight dieting women independent of diet and activity. Obesity (Silver Spring) 2008;16:2481–2488.
6.	Sauvant MP, Pepin D. Drinking water and cardiovascular disease. Food Chem Toxicol. 2002;40:1311–25.

7. Hatton DC, Yue Q, McCarron DA. Mechanisms of calcium's effects on blood pressure. Semin Nephrol. 1995 Nov;15(6):593-602.

8. Turlapaty, P.D.; Altura, B.M. Magnesium deficiency produces spasms of coronary arteries: Relationship to etiology of sudden death ischemic heart disease. Science 1980, 208, 198–200.

9. M. Girona, E. K. Grasser, A. G. Dulloo and J. P. Montani. Cardiovascular and metabolic responses to tap water ingestion in young humans: does the water temperature matter? Acta Physiol 2014, 211, 358–370.

10. Chang C.C., Ho S.C., Tsai S.S., Yang C.Y. Ischemic heart disease mortality reduction in an arseniasis-endemic area in southwestern Taiwan after a switch in the tap-water supply system. J. Toxicol. Environ. Health A. 2004;67:1353–1361.

93. OBESITY

Introduction

Obesity is a global problem.[1] According to the Centers for Disease Control and Prevention, obesity can be diagnosed from the Body Mass Index (BMI), which is a person's weight in kilograms divided by the square of the body height in meters.[2] According to them, underweight refers to a BMI of less than 18.5, normal to a BMI of 18.5 to <25, overweight to a BMI of 25.0 to <30, and obese to a BMI of 30.0 or higher. They further define obesity as Class 1: if the BMI is 30 to < 35; Class 2: if the BMI is 35 to < 40 and Class 3 ("extreme" or "severe" obesity) if the BMI of 40 or higher. Obesity is associated with a plethora of health problems, including osteoarthritis, gall bladder disease, hyperuricemia, gout, non-alcoholic fatty liver, several forms of cancer, back pain, and depression.[3] It is also associated with, hypertension, dyslipidemia, diabetes, metabolic syndrome and obstructive sleep apnea - conditions that increase cardiovascular risk, and lead to an increase in cardiovascular morbidity and mortality.[4]

Scientific Evidence

- The higher the BMI, the higher the systolic and diastolic blood pressure. It is estimated that almost 78 percent of primary hypertension in men and 65 percent in women can be ascribed to excess weight.[5] Clinical studies indicate that maintenance of a BMI < 25 is helpful in preventing the development of high blood pressure. Weight loss helps reduce blood pressure in those already suffering from hypertension.[6]
- Overweight and obese people have several times the normal risk of developing diabetes mellitus.[7] This also applies to children and adolescents.
- Obesity is associated with a marked increase in ischemic heart disease and stroke. Obese children and obese adolescents face a twofold or higher risk of suffering from hypertension, coronary heart disease, and stroke, during adulthood.[8] Obesity increases the risk of depression.[9] Depression is a risk factor for cardiovascular diseases.

- Obesity is associated with an increase in abdominal (visceral) fat, which results in increased inflammation, insulin resistance, and endothelial dysfunction.
- Obesity is associated with a marked increase in cardiovascular mortality.[10] Being overweight or obese in middle age shortens life expectancy by an estimated 4–7 years.[11]

Conclusion

Obesity is associated with significant morbidity and premature mortality. Obesity is unfortunately on the rise. Evidence based data shows striking improvement in cardiovascular risk factors with weight reduction. There is also a significant reduction in cardiovascular morbidity and mortality.

Lifestyle Implications

Monitor your weight and keep your BMI within the normal range. Maintaining normal weight will help you live healthier and longer, with a significant reduction in your risk of suffering from cardiovascular diseases or a premature cardiovascular death.

References

1. Hruby A, Hu FB. The Epidemiology of Obesity: A Big Picture. PharmacoEconomics. 2015;33(7):673-689.
2. https://www.cdc.gov/obesity/adult/defining.html
3. Must A, Spadano J, Coakley EH, Field AE, et al. The disease burden associated withoverweight and obesity. JAMA. 1999;282:1523-1529.
4. Zalesin K.C., Franklin B.A., Miller W.M., et al. Impact of obesity on cardiovascular disease. Med. Clin. North Am. 2011;95:919–937.
5. Garrison RJ, Kannel WB, Stokes J, III, Castelli WP. Incidence and precursors of hypertension in young adults: the Framingham Offspring Study. Prev Med. 1987;16:235–251.
6. Stevens VJ, Obarzanek E, Cook NR, et al. Long-term weight loss and changes in blood pressure: results of the Trials of Hypertension Prevention, phase II. Ann Intern Med. 2001;134:1–11.
7. Abdullah A, Peeters A, de Courten M, Stoelwinder J. The magnitude of association between overweight and obesity and the risk of diabetes: A meta-analysis of prospective cohort studies. Diabetes Res Clin Pract. 2010 Sep;89(3):309–19.
8. Reilly JJ, Kelly J. Long-term impact of overweight and obesity in childhood and adolescence on morbidity and premature mortality in adulthood: systematic review. Int J Obes. 2011 Jul;35(7):891–8.

9. Floriana S. Luppino, MD; Leonore M. de Wit, et al. Overweight, Obesity, and Depression. A Systematic Review and Meta-analysis of Longitudinal Studies. Arch Gen Psychiatry. 2010;67(3):220-229.

10. Chen Y, Copeland WK, Vedanthan R, Grant E, Lee JE, Gu D, et al. Association between body mass index and cardiovascular disease mortality in east Asians and south Asians: pooled analysis of prospective data from the Asia Cohort Consortium. BMJ. 2013 Oct 1;347: f5446–f5446. oct01 1.

11. Peeters A, Barendregt JJ, Willekens F, Mackenbach JP, Al Mamun A, Bonneux L, et al. Obesity in adulthood and its consequences for life expectancy: a life-table analysis. Ann Intern Med. 2003 Jan 7;138(1):24–32.

94. WEIGHT LOSS SURGERY

Introduction

Obesity is associated with an increased incidence of many diseases, including asthma, weight-bearing degenerative problems, several forms of cancer, and depression.[1] It is also associated with hypertension, dyslipidemia, diabetes, and obstructive sleep apnea - conditions that increase cardiovascular risk, resulting in an increase in cardiovascular morbidity and mortality.[2] Bariatric surgery is an extremely effective method of weight loss.[3] The resultant beneficial effects on health are numerous,[4] including a dramatic decrease in cardiovascular risk factors.[5] In 1991, the National Institutes of Health suggested that surgical therapy is appropriate if there is morbid obesity (BMI>40) or if the BMI is >35 in the presence of significant comorbidities.[6]

Scientific Evidence

- Bariatric surgery helps reduce both systolic blood pressure (by 4–15 mmHg) and diastolic blood pressure (by 2-5 mmHg) after 1–2 years. Some patients notice a complete resolution of their high blood pressure.[7]
- Bariatric surgery improves the lipid profile with decreases in low-density lipoprotein cholesterol and triglyceride levels and increases in the high-density lipoprotein cholesterol levels.[8]
- Diabetes and insulin resistance are dramatically improved after bariatric surgery, often preceeding a significant weight loss.[9] Up to 80% of diabetic patients develop a normal glycemic profile within a year or two and about 36% remain free of diabetes, 10-year post-surgery.[7]
- Obesity, is an inflammatory state. Inflammatory markers show a significant decrease following gastric banding or gastric bypass surgery.[10] There is also a significant improvement in obstructive sleep apnea.[11]
- Post-surgery, these patients have a reduced progression of atherosclerosis.[12] There are also favorable changes in cardiac geometry following bariatric surgery in both adults and adolescents, with the left ventricular mass decreased by 25–30 grams and left atrial volume being reduced by 6–15 ml.[13]

- There is a marked reduction in cardiac events,[7] and cardiovascular related deaths following bariatric surgery.[14]

Conclusion

Obesity is associated with significant morbidity and premature mortality. Evidence based data indicates a striking improvement in cardiovascular risk factors with bariatric surgery. There is also a significant reduction in cardiovascular morbidity and mortality.

Lifestyle Implications

Consider bariatric surgery if your BMI is over 40 or if your BMI is over 35 in the presence of significant comorbidities – and you are unable to lose weight by other means. It will help decrease your risk of premature cardiovascular disease or death.

References

1. Must A, Spadano J, Coakley EH, Field AE, et al. The disease burden associated withoverweight and obesity. JAMA. 1999;282:1523-1529.
2. Zalesin K.C., Franklin B.A., Miller W.M., et al. Impact of obesity on cardiovascular disease. Med. Clin. North Am. 2011;95:919–937.
3. Sjostrom L, Lindroos AK, Peltonen M, et al. Lifestyle, diabetes, and cardiovascular risk factors 10 years after bariatric surgery. N Engl J Med. 2004 Dec 23;351(26):2683–93.
4. Karmali S, Stoklossa CJ, Sharma A, et al. Bariatric surgery: A primer. Canadian Family Physician. 2010;56(9):873-879.
5. Williams DB, Hagedorn JC, Lawson EH, et al. Gastric bypass reduces biochemical cardiac risk factors. Surg Obes Relat Dis. 2007 Jan-Feb;3(1):8–13.
6. National Institutes of Health Consensus Development Panel. Gastrointestinal surgery for severe obesity. Ann Intern Med. 1991;115:956-961.
7. Sjostrom L, Lindroos AK, Peltonen M, et al. Lifestyle, diabetes, and cardiovascular risk factors 10 years after bariatric surgery. N Engl J Med. 2004 Dec 23;351(26):2683–93.
8. Benraoune F, Litwin SE. Reductions in Cardiovascular Risk After Bariatric Surgery. Current opinion in cardiology. 2011;26(6):555-561.
9. Pories WJ, Swanson MS, MacDonald KG, et al. Who would have thought it? an operation proves to be the most effective therapy for adult-onset diabetes mellitus. Ann Surg. 1995;222:339-352.
10. Brethauer SA, Heneghan HM, Eldar S, et al. Early effects of gastric bypass on endothelial function, inflammation, and cardiovascular risk in obese patients. Surg Endosc. 2011 Mar 17.

11. Henry Buchwald, Yoav Avidor, Eugene Braunwald, et al. Bariatric Surgery: A Systematic Review and Meta-analysis. JAMA. 2004;292(14):1724-1737.

12. Buchwald H, Varco RL, Matts JP, et al. Effect of partial ileal bypass surgery on mortality and morbidity from coronary heart disease in patients with hypercholesterolemia. Report of the Program on the Surgical Control of the Hyperlipidemias (POSCH) N Engl J Med. 1990 Oct 4;323(14):946–55.

13. Owan T, Avelar E, Morley K, Jiji R, et al. Favorable changes in cardiac geometry and function following gastric bypass surgery: 2-year follow-up in the Utah obesity study. J Am Coll Cardiol. 2011 Feb 8;57(6):732–9.

14. Sjostrom L, Narbro K, Sjostrom CD, et al. Effects of bariatric surgery on mortality in Swedish obese subjects. N Engl J Med. 2007 Aug 23;357(8):741–52.

95. WINE

Introduction

The cardiovascular benefits of drinking an alcoholic beverage in moderate amounts have been well documented. Moderate drinking refers to drinking one to two drinks per day for men and one drink per day for women. A drink is represented by one 12 oz. beer, 4 oz. of wine, 1.5 oz. of 80-proof spirits, or 1 oz. of 100-proof spirits. Fermented drinks were imbibed almost 10,000 years ago by the humans during the Neolithic period, and their health benefits touted. Recently, it was noted that despite having similar intakes of animal fats, French people had half the coronary heart disease death rate when compared to Americans. This "French Paradox" was attributed to the very high intake of red wine by the French.[1] Wine is made from grape skins, juice and seeds. Resveratrol is produced by the grape vine as a defence against fungal infections, and is present in the grape skin. Red wine is made from dark colored grapes, with the red color coming from anthocyan pigments (also called anthocyanins), a beneficial falvanoid present in the skin of these grapes. Anthocyanins and resveratrol are antioxidants, and confer additional protective effect, besides that obtained from the alcohol, in protecting against cardiovascular diseases.[2] Pharmacological properties of anthocyanins include anti-inflammatory, vasodilatatory, and free radicals scavenging activity - activities that result in cardioprotection.[3] White wine is made from the pulp of grapes and usually does not include the skin, and therefore lacks both resveratrol and anthocyanins. Vaso-relaxation is also induced by another phenolic compound called procyanidin, present in the red wine.4Wines also contain helpful non-flavonoids compounds such as hydroxycinnamic acid, benzoic acid, tannins and stilbenes.

Scientific Evidence

- In a study of mortality in 18 developed countries, researchers suggested that a reduced mortality appeared to be related to drinking of red wine.[5]
- In a study involving 13,000 individuals, wine drinkers had a decreased coronary risk, when compared to beer and spirit drinkers.[6]

- A recent meta-analysis of eight studies on wine and beer consumption and cardiovascular risk demonstrated that wine-drinkers exhibited almost 32% less cardiovascular disease when compared with nondrinkers.[7]
- Several reviews have confirmed the beneficial effects of moderate wine consumption on cardiovascular health, and this protection is more than that obtained by consuming other alcoholic drinks.[8-10]

Conclusion

Mild to moderate alcohol drinking is cardioprotective. This means an average of one to two drinks per day for men and one drink per day for women. (A drink is one 12 oz. beer, 4 oz. of wine, 1.5 oz. of 80-proof spirits, or 1 oz. of 100-proof spirits.) The benefits occur from alcohol induced increases in the high-density lipoprotein cholesterol, a reduction in low-density lipoprotein cholesterol oxidation, vasodilatation and several anti-clotting effects. Drinking red wine confers a further advantage because of the antioxidant effects generated by the polyphenols that are present in the skin of the dark colored grapes.

Lifestyle Implications

A glass of red wine a day keeps your heart healthy – and the heart doctor away.

References

1   Renaud S, de Lorgeril M. Wine, alcohol, platelets, and the French paradox for coronary heart disease. Lancet. 1992;339:1523–6

2   Huxley RR, Neil HA. The relation between dietary flavonol intake and coronary heart disease mortality: A meta-analysis of prospective cohort studies. Eur J Clin Nutr. 2003;57:904–8.

3   Marcello Iriti, Mara Rossoni, Michele Borgo et al. Benzothiadiazole Enhances Resveratrol and Anthocyanin Biosynthesis in Grapevine, Meanwhile Improving Resistance to Botrytis cinereal. J. Agric. Food Chem. 2004, 52, 4406–4413

4   Vidavalur R, Otani H, Singal PK, Maulik N. Significance of wine and resveratrol in cardiovascular disease: French paradox revisited. Experimental & Clinical Cardiology. 2006;11(3):217-225.

5   St Leger AS, Cochrane AL, Moore F. Factors associated with cardiac mortality in developed countries with particular reference to the consumption of wine. Lancet. 1979;1:1017–20.

6   Gronbaek M, Tjonneland A, Johansen D, Stripp C, Overvad K. Type of alcohol and drinking pattern in 56,970 Danish men and women. Eur J Clin Nutr. 2000;54:174–6.

7   Huxley RR, Neil HA. The relation between dietary flavonol intake and coronary heart disease mortality: A meta-analysis of prospective cohort studies. Eur J Clin Nutr. 2003;57:904–8.

8   Liberale L, Bonaventura A, Montecucco F, Dallegri F, Carbone F. Impact of Red Wine Consumption on Cardiovascular Health. Curr Med Chem. 2017 May 17.

9   Lippi G, Franchini M, Favaloro EJ, Targher G. Moderate red wine consumption and cardiovascular disease risk: beyond the "French paradox". Semin Thromb Hemost. 2010 Feb;36(1):59-70.

10   Arranz S, Chiva-Blanch G, Valderas-Martínez P, Medina-Remón A, Lamuela-Raventós RM, Estruch R. Wine, Beer, Alcohol and Polyphenols on Cardiovascular Disease and Cancer. Nutrients. 2012;4(7):759-781.

Introduction

Working more than the standard work week may be detrimental to the physical and mental health of humans.[1] There is an associated negative impact on social and family life. The quality of life is also affected.[2] The health damage also involves the cardiovascular system.[3] and appears to be dose related. Sudden death in Japanese overtime workers has been termed as Karoshi and is attributed to the cardiovascular system.[4]

Scientific Evidence

- An increase in working hours is associated with an increase in hypertension. A study looked at 1,079 subjects, with average working time of 47.68 hours per week. The proportion of overtime workers was 61.0% (cutoff of 40 hours per week). In this study, as the number of overtime hours increased, so did the diagnosis of hypertension.[5]
- A study of 2,194 workers indicate that those working more than 50 hours overtime per month in Japan, had a 3.7 times higher risk of non-insulin dependant diabetes mellitus after controlling for known risk factors.[6]
- Another study found that working more than 10 hours/day resulted in an increased risk of metabolic syndrome among Japanese male workers.[7] Metabolic syndrome is closely associated with cardiovascular disease, myocardial infarction, stroke, and all-cause mortality.
- A meta-analysis of 11 studies have confirmed that long working hours were associated with an increased risk of cardiovascular disease.[8]
- A retrospective cohort study of 1,926 individuals from the Panel Study of Income Dynamics, revealed that increasing work week was associated with a dose-related increased risk of cardiovascular disease. These employees were employed for at least 10 years and were studied from1986 to 2011.
- Long working hours are also related to an increase in several other cardiovascular risk factors, including decreased physical activity, increased smoking, and increased stress and depression.[9]

- Evaluation of Karoshi or deaths attritubed to overwork in Japan revealed that over 70% of the sudden deaths were due to a sudden stroke or a fatal cardiac event.[10]
- These excess working hours related risk factors affect several neurohormonal systems in the human body leading to an increased risk of cardiovascular diseases and mortality.

Conclusion

Scientific data is clear that working extra hours every week are detrimental for health, especially cardiovascular. The effect appears to be linear – the more hours worked overtime – the higher the risk of cardiovascular events or death.

Lifestyle Implications.

Thinks twice before working overtime. It may save your life.

References

1. Tarumi K, Hagihara A, Morimoto K. A prospective observation of onsets of health defects associated with working hours. Ind Health. 2003;41:101–108.
2. Maruyama S, Morimoto K. Effects of long workhours on life-style, stress and quality of life among intermediate Japanese managers. Scand J Work Environ Health 1996;22(5):353-359.
3. Virtanen M, Ferrie JE, Singh-Manoux A, et al. Overtime work and incident coronary heart disease: The Whitehall II prospective cohort study. Eur Heart J. 2010;31:1737–1744.
4. Ke DS. Overwork, stroke, and karoshi-death from overwork. Acta Neurol Taiwan. 2012 Jun;21(2):54-9.
5. Yoo DH, Kang M, Paek D, Min B, Cho S. Effect of Long Working Hours on Self reported Hypertension among Middle-aged and Older Wage Workers. Annals of Occupational and Environmental Medicine. 2014;26:25.
6. Kawakami N, Araki S, Takatsuka N, Shimizu H, Ishibashi H. Overtime, psychosocial working conditions, and occurrence of non- insulin dependent diabetes mellitus in Japanese men. Journal of Epidemiology and Community Health. 1999;53(6):359-363.
7. Kobayashi T, Suzuki E, Takao S, Doi H. Long working hours and metabolic syndrome among Japanese men: a cross-sectional study. BMC Public Health. 2012;12:395.

8. Kang MY, Park H, Seo JC, et al. Long working hours and cardiovascular disease: a meta-analysis of epidemiologic studies. J Occup Environ Med. 2012 May;54(5):532-7.

9. Virtanen M, Stansfeld SA, Fuhrer R, Ferrie JE, Kivimäki M. Overtime work as a predictor of major depressive episode: A 5-year follow-up of the Whitehall II study. PloS One. 2012;7: e30719.

10. Ke DS. Overwork, stroke, and karoshi-death from overwork. Acta Neurol Taiwan. 2012 Jun;21(2):54-9.

97. YOGA: ASANAS

Introduction

Yoga evolved over thousands of years in India. It has become an important activty for maintaining proper physical and mental health, in otherwise healthy individuals. Its popularity in the general public has been accompanied by an unprejudiced curiosity in the scientific community. A plethora of properly designed human studies have emerged, documenting that yoga poses trigger several neuro-endocrine and hemodynamic changes that beneficially modify the initiation and/or progression of several disease processes. This includes cardiovascular diseases. The popularity of yoga in the US is growing rapidly, and recent estimates indicate that almost 9.5% of U.S. adults (21 million) practiced yoga in 2012.[1] Yoga asanas are physical exercises that improve flexibility and strength. They use the body's weight and the earth's gravity to achieve a wide range of poses.

Scientific Evidence

- Yoga asanas reduce high blood pressure, obesity, hypercholesterolemia, diabetes mellitus, smoking and inactivity.[2] Inflammatory markers are reduced and there is an increase in the parasympathetic activity. These positive modulations suggest a potential role in the primary prevention of coronary artery disease. In patients with established disease, yoga may help prevent future events.[3] Studies have also reported a regression in coronary atherosclerosis.[4] Yoga also improves functionality as well as mentation in patients following a heart attack and can play an important role in cardiac rehabilitation.[5]

- Yoga practice in several studies have shown to help patients in smoking cessation.

- Yoga asanas, result in a significant improvement in overall physical health, endurance, strength, flexibility, posture and balance.

- A yogic lifestyle also result in weight loss, with significant reduction in cardiovascular risk.[6]

- In a recent meta-analytic review of 17 studies (22 trials), yoga was associated with a clinically significant decline in both systolic and diastolic blood pressure (−4.17 and −3.26 mmHg, respectively).[7]

- Yoga may play a complementary role in reducing the risks associated with prediabetes and diabetes. Yoga is beneficial even if the diabetes is poorly controlled, or burdened with complications.

- Many studies have reported that yoga improves lipid profiles in not only healthy individuals, but also in patients with hypertension, diabetes and established coronary artery disease.

- Regular practice of yoga reduces inflammation as it lowers basal TNF-α, IL-6 levels, and C-reactive protein levels – all biomarkers of inflammation.

- Yoga has been reported to decrease perceived stress and reactivity to stressors, enhance stress-related coping, reduce symptoms of depression and anxiety, decrease anger, tension and fatigue, enhance psychological well-being, and reduce sleep disturbances. Overall, well-being is better in yoga practitioners, with most experiencing a better quality of life.

- Yoga has also shown benefits in the population needing cardiac rehabilitation. Yoga improves many physical and mental parameters in stroke patients. The beneficial effects of yoga in stroke patients include improvement in flexibility, muscle strength, fatigue and balance. There is also a a decrease in stress, anxiety, and depression, in these patients.

Conclusion

Several randomized controlled clinical trials confirms the therapeutic benefits of yoga in cardiovascular diseases, when it is used as a complementary modality. Yoga asanas can be performed anywhere, require no special equipment, are gentle on the joints and can be modified for each person. Yoga uses the body and gravity as resistance, preventing excessive impact. Yoga is simple to follow and cost-effective with a high compliance rate. Yoga has few side effects, and the risk of serious injury is quite low.

Lifestyle Implications

The evidence based data on the adjunctive therapeutic benefit of yoga asanas in cardiovascular diseases is well established and is extremely persuasive. Join a yoga class today.

References

1. NCCIH: https://nccih.nih.gov/research/statistics/NHIS/2012/mind-body/yoga; accessed October 21, 2015.
2. Tulpule TH, Shah HM, Shah SJ, et al. Yogic exercises in the management of ischaemic heart disease. Indian Heart Journal. 1971;23(4):259–264.
3. Lau HL, Kwong JS, Yeung F, et al. Yoga for secondary prevention of coronary heart disease. Cochrane Database Syst Rev. 2012 Dec 12;12:CD009506.
4. Yogendra J, Yogendra H, Ambardekar S, et al. Beneficial effects of yoga lifestyle on reversibility of ischaemic heart disease: Caring Heart Project of International Board of Yoga. JAPI. 2004; 52:283.
5. Gomes-Neto M, Rodrigues-Jr ES, Silva-Jr WM et al. Effects of Yoga in Patients with Chronic Heart Failure: A Meta-Analysis. Arq Bras Cardiol. 2014 Nov;103(5):433-439.
6. Damodaran A, Malathi A, Patil N, et al. Therapeutic potential of yoga practices in modifying cardiovascular risk profile in middle aged men and women. J Assoc Physicians India. 2002; 50:633–40.
7. Hagins M, States R, Selfe T, et al. Effectiveness of Yoga for Hypertension: Systematic Review and Meta-Analysis Evidence-Based Complementary and Alternative Medicine. Volume 2013 (2013), Article ID 649836, 13 pages.

98. YOGA: PRANAYAMA

Introduction

Yoga evolved over thousands of years in India. Besides putting the body through a wide variety of poses, yoga practice also involves a period of controlled breathing exercises, called pranayama. The latter has been the focus of several scientific studies, with results documenting significant beneficial effects on the pulmonary function, both in healthy individuals, and those with respiratory diseases. Evidence based data reveals health benefits in many non-respiratory conditions also, and this includes cardiovascular diseases.[1] There are many types of yogic pranayama techniques, but in general, the slow type of breathing exercises appear to have more beneficial effects on the prevention and management of cardiovascular disorders.[2] The popularity of yoga exercises in the US is growing rapidly, and recent estimates indicate that almost 9.5% of U.S. adults (21 million) practiced yoga in 2012.

Scientific Evidence

- Pranayama helps reduce blood pressure, both systolic and diastolic.[3]
- Several pranayama exercises increase the para-sympthatetic tone and help reduce the heart rate.[4]
- Several breathing modalities improve cardiovascular parameters in healthy as well as those with established coronary artery disease.[5] Practicing pranayama regularly for more than three months results in significant improvements in major parameters of lung function, in patients with coronary artery disease.
- Yoga also reduces stress and anxiety. Benefits are also noted in depression.[6]
- Patients after a heart attack achieved higher work rates and decreased their oxygen consumption, with controlled yogic breathing.[7]
- Yogic breathing exercises may also calm the electrical activity in the heart and help prevent irregular heart beats.[8]

Conclusion

Pranayama exercises are usually practiced along with yoga asanas and meditation. Most clinical studies include all three and benefits are often difficult to attribute to a paticular modality. However, some studies have focused on pranayama alone, and evidence based data indicates that these exercises improve lung function in healthy individuals as well as those with cardiovascular diseases. They also help alter the autonomic balance, with an increase in the parasympathetic tone. This increase helps reduce blood pressure and heart rate, changes that are cardiovascular friendly. Regularly performed, yogic breathing exercises also help mitigate stress, depression and anxiety.

Lifestyle Implications

The evidence based data on the adjunctive therapeutic benefit of yogic breathing exercises in cardiovascular diseases is encouraging. Pranayama exercises have no known side effects, require no infrastructure or costs and can easily be practiced anywhere, even by the chronically ill and the elderly. Practice pranayama – you will breathe better.

References

1. Bhavanani AB, Sanjay Z, Madanmohan. Immediate effect of sukha pranayama on cardiovascular variables in patients of hypertension. Int J Yoga Therap. 2011;(21):73-6.
2. Nivethitha L, Mooventhan A, Manjunath N. Effects of Various Prāṇāyāma on Cardiovascular and Autonomic Variables. Ancient Science of Life. 2016;36(2):72-77.
3. Singh S, Gaurav V, Parkash V. Effects of a 6-week nadi-shodhana pranayama training on cardio-pulmonary parameters. Journal of Physical Education and Sports Management. 2011;2:44–7.
4. Ashish Chaddha. Slow breathing and cardiovascular disease. Int J Yoga. 2015 Jul-Dec; 8(2).
5. Asha Yadav, Savita Singh, KP Singh, and Preeti Pai. Effect of yoga regimen on lung functions including diffusion capacity in coronary artery disease patients: A randomized controlled study. Int J Yoga. 2015 Jan-Jun; 8(1): 62–67.
6. Brown R.P., Gerbarg P.L., Sudarshan Kriya. Yogic breathing in the treatment of stress, anxiety, and depression. J Altern Complement Med. 2005; 11:711-717.
7. Telles S, Naveen KV. Yoga for rehabilitation: An overview. Indian J Med Sciences 1997; 51:123–127.

8. Dabhade AM, Pawar BH, Ghunage MS, Ghunage VM. Effect of pranayama (breathing exercise) on arrhythmias in the human heart. Explore (NY). 2012 Jan-Feb;8(1):12-5.

99. YOGA: MEDITATION

Introduction

Meditation, a mind body practice, was mentioned in Hindu scriptures around 1500 BC. It has been described as a process of contemplation, concentration, and reflection, leading to a state of inner calmness and physical relaxation. It has become a potentially important tool for improving individual health and wellness.[1] Benefits include improvements in several mental health ailments including insomnia, irritable bowel syndrome, symptoms related to premenstrual syndrome and menopause, and chronic pain. Its practice has also shown to be beneficial in several cardiovascular disorders.[2] It is generally easy to learn and safe to practice.

Scientific Evidence

- Several psychological states increase the risk of cardiovascular disease and mortality. These include anxiety, hostility, and depression. Meditation helps reduce the severity of these psychological risk factors.[3]
- In 56 pre-hypertensive men and women, patients practicing meditation exhibited a 4.8 mmHg reduction in systolic blood pressure and a 1.9 mmHg reduction in diastolic blood pressure.[4]
- Meditation helps reduce blood pressure in patients with established hypertension. In a large meta-analysis of 9 randomized controlled trials, researchers found that a transcendental meditation program lowered systolic blood pressure by an average of 4.7 mmHg and diastolic blood pressure by an average of 3.2 mmHg, when compared with control groups.[5]
- Meditation reduces type 2 diabetes. Sixteen weeks of transcendental meditation in 103 subjects with stable coronary heart disease, there was an improvement in insulin resistance. A decrease in postprandial blood sugar rise was also noted in 50 patients with type 2 diabetes.[6]
- Meditation improves the lipid profile. Cooper and associates noted a 10% reduction in total cholesterol in patients who practiced meditation for 13 months.[7]
- Meditation is helpful in reducing the metabolic syndrome, especially in African Americans.[8]

- Several large reviews have documented that meditation reduces cardiovascular mortality. A meta-analysis of 23 randomized controlled trials evaluating a total of 3,180 participants, meditation improved outcomes among patients with coronay heart disease.[9] In another meta-analysis of 37 studies, meditation programs resulted in a 29% reduction in recurrence of myocardial infarction, and a 34% reduction in cardiac mortality - in patients with established coronary heart disease.[10]

Conclusion

Evidence based data confirms that meditation improves many risk factors for cardiovascular diseases including hypertension, type 2 diabetes mellitus, dyslipidemia, and high cortisol levels. Meditative practices also reduce cardiovascular morbidity and mortality.

Lifestyle Implications

Meditate! It will not only calm your brain but also help your heart.

References

1. Sharma H. Meditation: Process and effects. Ayu. 2015;36(3):233-237.
2. Ray I. B. et al. Meditation and coronary heart disease: a review of the current clinical evidence. Ochsner J 14, 696–703 (2014).
3. Leite JR, Ornellas FL, Amemiya TM, et al. Effect of progressive self-focus meditation on attention, anxiety, and depression scores. Percept Mot Skills. 2010 Jun;110(3 Pt 1):840–848.
4. Hughes JW, Fresco DM, Myerscough R, van Dulmen MH, Carlson LE, Josephson R. Randomized controlled trial of mindfulness-based stress reduction for prehypertension. Psychosom Med. 2013 Oct;75(8):721–728.
5. Anderson JW, Liu C, Kryscio RJ. Blood pressure response to transcendental meditation: a meta-analysis. Am J Hypertens. 2008 Mar;21(3):310–316.
6. Chaiopanont S. Hypoglycemic effect of sitting breathing meditation exercise on type 2 diabetes at Wat Khae Nok Primary Health Center in Nonthaburi province. J Med Assoc Thai. 2008 Jan;91(1):93–98.
7. Cooper MJ, Aygen MM. A relaxation technique in the management of hypercholesterolemia. J Human Stress. 1979 Dec;5(4):24–27.
8. Vaccarino V, Kondwani KA, Kelley ME, et al. Effect of meditation on endothelial function in Black Americans with metabolic syndrome: a randomized trial. Psychosom Med. 2013 Jul-Aug;75(6):591–599.
9. Linden W, Stossel C, Maurice J. Psychosocial interventions for patients with coronary artery disease: a meta-analysis. Arch Intern Med. 1996 Apr

8;156(7):745–752. Erratum in: Arch Intern Med. 1996 Nov 11;156(20):2302.

10. Dusseldorp E, van Elderen T, Maes S, Meulman J, Kraaij V. A meta-analysis of psychoeducational programs for coronary heart disease patients. Health Psychol. 1999 Sep;18(5):506–519.

Introduction

Walking is a normal human activity. It is the main method for locomotion in most legged animals. Walking speed in humans depends on a lot of factors and averages about 3 miles per hour. Walking involves contractions of various skeletal muscles via continuous bodily movements, resulting in an increase in blood circulation and energy expenditure. A sedentary lifestyle increases cardiovascular disease and regular walking can help mitigate this modifiable risk.[1]

Scientific Evidence

- Based on a meta-analysis of 12 studies, involving 295,177 participants free of coronary heart disease at baseline, Zheng and colleagues found that 8 MET (metabolic equivalent of task) hours/week of walking (approximately 30 minutes/day, 5 days/week) was associated with a 19% reduction in coronary heart disease risk.[2]

- A quicker walking pace and a higher walking volume were associated with more cardiovascular protection.[3]

- In patients with established cardiovascular disease, walking conferred protection against death. This was noted in a study of 837 men and women, followed for an average of 5.6 years. During this period, there were 175 deaths. Walkers had a decreased incidence of death.[4]

- In a larger study of 23,747 men and women with and without metabolic abnormalities (abnormal blood pressure, low high-density lipoprotein cholesterol, diabetes mellitus, increased waist circumference, and low-grade inflammation as evidenced by a C-reactive protein $\geq$ 3 mg/L), researchers found that low dose physical activity was cardiovascular protective.[5]

- Walking as a physical activity reduces cardiovascular risk via several beneficial mechanisms, including reduction in inflammation, triglycerides and diastolic blood pressure, and an improvement in dyslipidemia and high-density lipoprotein cholesterol levels.

- Walking briskly for at least 30 minutes per day also improves insulin sensitivity and glycemic control, reducing the risk of type 2 diabetes.[6]
- Walking is a physical activity that can help weight loss and improve several emotions that are detrimental to the cardiovascular system, such as depression.

Conclusion

Sedentary behaviors, such as television viewing, driving in a car, or sitting, are associated with an increase in cardiovascular diseases, both in men, and women. The American Heart Association recommends at least 150 minutes of moderate exercise per week or 75 minutes of vigorous exercise per week (or a combination of moderate and vigorous activity) for cardiovascular protection.[7] Walking may help satisfy some of these goals. Pedometers are cheap and easy to use. They can help monitor and achieve walking related exercise - aim for a minimum of 3000 steps in 30 minutes on 5 days each week.[8]

Lifestyle Implications

Leisure time walking is an easy and effective evidence-based exercise modality for cardiovascular disease prevention. Take a daily walk outside and admire nature!

References

1. Murtagh EM, Murphy MH, Boone-Heinonen J. Walking – the first steps in cardiovascular disease prevention. Current opinion in cardiology. 2010;25(5):490-496.
2. Zheng H, Orsini N, Amin J, et al. Quantifying the dose-response of walking in reducing coronary heart disease risk: meta-analysis. Eur J Epidemiol. 2009;24:181–92.
3. Hamer M, Chida Y. Walking and primary prevention: a meta-analysis of prospective cohort studies. Br J Sports Med. 2008;42:238–43.
4. Hamer M, Stamatakis E. Physical activity and mortality in men and women with diagnosed cardiovascular disease. Eur J Cardiovasc Prev Rehabil. 2009;16:156–60.
5. Hamer M, Stamatakis E. Low-dose physical activity attenuates cardiovascular disease mortality in men and women with clustered metabolic risk factors. Circ Cardiovasc Qual Outcomes. 2012 Jul 1;5(4):494-9.
6. Hidetaka Hamasaki. Daily physical activity and type 2 diabetes: A review. World J Diabetes 2016 June 25; 7(12): 243-251.

7. http://www.heart.org/HEARTORG/HealthyLiving/PhysicalActivity/Fit
    nessBasics/American-Heart-Association-Recommendations-for-Physical-
    Activity-in-Adults_UCM_307976_Article.jsp#.WQy7lOXys1I (accessed
    May 5, 2017).
8. Marshall S, Levy S, Tudor-Locke C, et al. Translating Physical Activity
    Recommendations into a Pedometer-Based Step Goal 3000 Steps in 30
    Minutes. American Journal of Preventive Medicine. 2009;36:410–5.

101. WHOLE GRAINS

Introduction

A natural grain consists of an outer layer called the bran, a middle part called the endosperm and an inner part called the germ. The outer bran layer is composed of cellulose, hemicelluloses and arabinoxylan – these are essentially non-digestable, insoluble and poorly fermentable carbohydrates. They help protect the endosperm and the germ, from the hostile external environment - weather, insects, molds, and bacteria. The endosperm is mainly starch (50%-75%) and protein (8%–18 %). It also contains viscous soluble fibers, fermentable oligosaccharides, lignans, vitamins, minerals, polyphenols, oils, and other phytonutrients. It provides nourishment to the growing seedling. The germ represents the plant embryo and is a nutrient rich core. The refining process, removes the majority of bran and germ, resulting in a considerable loss of fiber, minerals, vitamins, and phytonutrients. White breads, white rice and white flour are all made from refined grains. Whole grains commonly consumed in the United States of American include wheat, rice, and maize, oats, rye, barley, triticale, sorghum, and millet. According to American Association of Cereal Chemists International, whole grains (in commercial food products) should contain bran, endosperm, and germ, in the same relative proportions as they exist in the intact grain, even after processing.[1] Oatmeal, quinoa, brown rice, rolled oats, bulgur, wild rice and popcorn are naturally whole grains. The health benefits of consuming whole grains have been known since Hippocrates (4th century BC). Major scientific studies during the past two decades, have shown several benefits of whole grain intake on human health, including cardiovascular health.

Scientific Evidence

- A pooled data from six cohort studies with 286,125 participants, the risk of developing diabetes decreased by 21% with a 2 serving/day increase in whole grain consumption. Improvements in insulin sensitivity were noted as early as 6 weeks after consumption of a whole grain diet – there was a 10% lower fasting insulin level and there was a 13% lower insulin resistance.[2] Reductions in fasting glucose, low-density lipoprotein cholesterol, total cholesterol, and body fat percentage, were also documented in two meta-analysis.

- Whole grain consumption is beneficial in preventing weight gain and obesity. One study estimated that for every 40 gram increase in daily whole grain intake, the weight gain is decreased by almost 2.4 lbs.[3]

- The association between whole grain intake and a reduction in cardiovascular disease has been well documented.[4] The reductions have been seen in hypertension, heart attacks, stroke and heart failure.

- Reductions in all-cause mortality has been noted in both men and women with an increased intake of whole grains in several epidemiological studies. In a recent meta-analysis of fourteen studies which included 786,076 participants and 23,957 cardiovascular deaths, an inverse relationship between whole grain intake and cardiovascular mortality was confirmed.[5]

Conclusion

Whole grains have significant benefits on cardiovascular health. The 2015 Dietary Guidelines for Americans,[6] recommend that all Americans age 9 and up, consume at least half of their grains as whole grains - this means eating 3 to 5 servings or more of whole grains every day. A serving is equivalent to: 1/2 cup cooked rice, pasta, or cooked cereal, one ounce of dry pasta, rice or other dry grain; 1 slice of bread, 1 small muffin (weighing one ounce) or 1 cup of ready-to-eat cereal flakes.[7] The protection is obtained from the bran and the germ which are retained in the whole grain products. Foods listing ingredients as 100% wheat or colored brown are not necessarily whole grains. Look for the Whole Grain stamp on the product from the Whole Grains Council or the word, 'whole' before the word grain in the ingredients.

Lifestyle Implications

Whole grains (at least 3 servings per day) should be eaten regularly — their ingestion is cardioprotective.

References

1. FDA:
   http://www.fda.gov/NewsEvents/Newsroom/PressAnnouncements/2006/ucm108598.htm
2. Pereira MA, Jacobs DR, Pins JJ, Raatz S, Gross M, Slavin J, Seaquist E. The effect of whole grains on insulin sensitivity in overweight hyperinsulinemic adults. Am J Clin Nutr 2002;75:848–55.
3. Seal CJ, Brownlee IA. Whole grains and health, evidence from observational and intervention studies. Cereal Chem. 2010;87:167–74.
4. Koh-Banerjee P, Franz M, Sampson L, Liu S, Jacobs DR, Jr, Spiegelman D, Willett W, Rimm E. Changes in whole-grain, bran, and cereal fiber consumption in relation to 8-y weight gain among men. Am J Clin Nutr 2004;80:1237–45.
5. Geng Zong, Alisa Gao, Frank B. Hu, and Qi Sun. Whole Grain Intake and Mortality from All Causes, Cardiovascular Disease, and Cancer: A Meta-analysis of Prospective Cohort Studies. Circulation, online June 13, 2016,
6. http://health.gov/dietaryguidelines/2015/guidelines/chapter-1/a-closer-look-inside-healthy-eating-patterns/#callout-wholegrains
7. http://wholegrainscouncil.org/whole-grains-101/us-dietary-guidelines-and-wg

Glossary

ACE: angiotensin converting enzyme – their inhibitors are common drugs that relax arteries and promote renal excretion of salt and water and help reduce blood pressure.

Adenopectin: a protein made by fat cells that plays a role in the development of insulin resistance and atherosclerosis.

Adipocyte: also known as lipocytes and fat cells that are specialized in storing energy as fat

Adrenal: glands found above the kidneys – they secrete a variety of hormones including adrenaline and the steroids aldosterone and cortisol

Adrenaline: hormone secreted by the adrenal glands in response to stress - increases heart rate, pulse rate, and blood pressure, and raises the blood levels of glucose and lipids.

Aerobic: occurring only in the presence of oxygen

Aggregability/ aggregation: the tendency or the process whereby the platelets clump together and form a clot

Algae: chlorophyll containing unicellular or multicellular organisms, present in fresh or salt water or moist ground

Angiogenesis: the growth of new blood vessels

Anthocyanins: red, purple, or blue pigment found in blueberries, cherries and plums and other colored vegetables and fruits – they are powerful antioxidants

Anthropometric: relating to measurements used to assess the size, shape and composition of the human body.

Antibodies: a blood protein produced by B cells as a primary immune defense. It is a response to and counteracting a specific antigen – usually an alien such as a virus or bacteria

Anticoagulants: substances that hinder coagulation of blood – could be a drug

Antioxidant: a substance that inhibits oxidation such as beta-carotene, vitamin C, and alpha-tocopherol

Anti-proliferative: retarding cell growth or spread

Aortic: relating to the aorta – the largest artery in the body arising from the top of the left ventricle which is the main pumping chamber of the heart

Apolipoprotein: proteins that bind lipids to form lipoproteins (and help transport the lipids)

Arrhythmia: an irregular or abnormal heart rhythm

Arterial: relating to an artery

Atherosclerosis: a silent process leading to the buildup of plaque inside the arteries and leading to narrowing and blockages – the usual cause of heart attacks, strokes, and peripheral vascular disease

Atherothrombotic: the formation of a blood clot within an artery, usually as a result of atherosclerotic lesion disruption

Atrial fibrillation: a fast and irregular heartbeat - may lead to blood clots, stroke, heart failure and other heart-related complications

Autoimmune: usually referred to an autoimmune disorder where the immune system attacks healthy cells in its own body by mistake

Autonomic nervous system: the nervous system that regulates the functions of the internal organs such as the heart, stomach and intestines

Bariatric surgery: weight loss surgery. The most common bariatric surgery procedures are gastric bypass, sleeve gastrectomy and adjustable gastric band

Baroreflex: feedback loop that plays an important role in short term blood pressure regulation

Bioactive: having an effect on a living tissue

Bioavailability: the degree and rate a substance is available for physiological activity – usually referred to an absorbed drug and the amount available in the body for bioactivity

Biomarker: a distinct biochemical, genetic, or molecular characteristic or substance that is an indicator of a particular biological condition or process

Bipolar: bipolar disease is a serious manic-depressive illness

Body Mass Index (BMI): a weight-to-height ratio - defines normal weight, overweight, and obesity in adults

Caffeine: a central nervous system stimulant found in coffee – it is the world's most widely consumed psychoactive drug

Calorie: the energy needed to raise the temperature of 1 gram of water through 1 °C – commonly used as a measurement of the amount of energy that food provides

Carbohydrates: substances such as sugar and starches that are major sources of energy for the human body

Carcinogens: a substance or agent capable of causing cancer

Cardiac rehabilitation: an outpatient medically supervised program of exercise and education for people following a heart attack, heart failure, heart valve surgery, coronary artery bypass grafting, or percutaneous coronary intervention

Cardiogenic: relating to the heart

Cardiomyopathy: a disease affecting the heart muscle – it causes the heart to become enlarged, thick, or stiff.

Cardiotoxicity: toxicity that affects the heart – may occur with cancer therapy

Cardiovascular: relating to the heart and blood vessels

Carotenoids: a group of pigments that are responsible for the bright red, yellow and orange colors of many fruits and vegetables

Cataracts: progressive opaqueness of the lens of the eyes – resulting in blurry or cloudy vision

Catecholamines: a group of sympathomimetic amines (including dopamine, epinephrine, and norepinephrine) that act as hormones and/or neurotransmitters

Cerebrovascular: relating to the brain and its blood vessels

Cholesterol: a steroid that's found in all cells of the body – high levels are associated with an increased risk for heart and blood vessel disease.

Chylomicron: a small lipoprotein particle – they transport exogenous cholesterol and triglycerides from the small intestine to the liver and adipose tissues

Circadian rhythm: an internal body clock – it regulates many physiological processes including when to sleep and when to rise

Cognitive: concerning mental processes such as perception, thinking, learning, and memory

Cohort: a group of individuals with something in common

Co-morbidity: the presence of two disorders or illnesses simultaneously or sequentially in the same patient

Congestive heart failure: failure of the heart to pump blood

COPD: Chronic Obstructive Pulmonary Disease – chronic obstruction of lung airflow interfering with normal breathing and not fully reversible

Coronary Artery Disease: disease (usually atherosclerosis) of the arteries that supply blood to the heart – the result may be angina or a heart attack

Coronary Heart Disease: heart diseases resulting from coronary artery narrowing or blockage

Cortisol: a steroid based hormone produced by the adrenal glands – it is also known as hydrocortisone

CRP: C-reactive protein – is a marker for inflammation in the body

Cytokines: a group of proteins (such as interferon, interleukin) that trigger inflammation

Dementia: a progressive condition characterized by multiple cognitive deficits. Alzheimer's disease accounts for 60 to 80 percent of cases.

Deoxyribonucleic acid: DNA – carries the genetic information for the transmission of hereditary traits

Diabetes Mellitus Type 2: a long-term metabolic disorder characterized by high blood sugar, insulin resistance, and relative lack of insulin – causes damage to the heart, eyes, kidneys, nerves, and other parts of the body.

Diastolic blood pressure: it indicates the pressure the blood is exerting against the walls of the arteries while the heart is resting between beats. If the blood pressure is 120/80, the diastolic pressure is 80 mm Hg (millimeters of mercury).

Dopamine: neurotransmitter; essential to the normal functioning of the central nervous system

Eclampsia: a life threatening high blood pressure complication during pregnancy – with one or more convulsions

Endogenous: produced internally

Endothelium: the single layer of cells lining the insides of the blood vessels, heart, and lymphatic vessels

Epidemiological: the incidence, distribution, and control of diseases in large populations

Epinephrine: also known as adrenaline – a hormone secreted by the adrenal gland. It is a stress hormone and causes increases in heart rate, pulse rate, and blood pressure, and raises the blood levels of glucose and lipids.

Ethanol: the intoxicating ingredient of alcoholic beverages – usually obtained from the fermentation of sugars and starches

Fibrinogen: a protein in the blood plasma that is changed into fibrin to form a blood clot

Flavanols/Flavanoid: plant based nutrients that have major antioxidant activities

Foam cells: macrophages (phagocytic white cells) laden with lipids – accumulating in the walls of the arteries and a part of the process of developing atherosclerosis

Gestational: period of fetal development from conception until birth

Glycated hemoglobin: is a form of hemoglobin that when measured gives the three-month average plasma glucose concentration - hemoglobin A1c, HbA1c, A1C, or Hb1c

Glycemic Index: a relative ranking of carbohydrate in foods according to how they affect blood glucose levels. Carbohydrate-containing foods can be classified as high- ($\geq$70), moderate- (56-69), or low-GI ($\leq$55) relative to pure glucose (GI=100). A low GI indicates a slow absorption

Growth hormone: also known as somatotropin is secreted by the pituitary and helps children grow and helps adults maintain tissues and organs

HDL: high density lipoprotein – the 'good cholesterol'. It carries the 'bad' LDL cholesterol away from the arteries and back to the liver

Hemodialysis: kidney dialysis – the process of purifying the blood, by removing fluid and waste products, from a person whose kidneys are not working normally

Hemorrhagic stroke: brain damage caused by a rupture of a weakened blood vessel – it is responsible for about 15% of all strokes

Hydrogenation: the process of converting liquid vegetable oils into solid or semi-solid fats, such as those present in margarine.

Hypercholesterolemia: high cholesterol levels in the blood

Hyperglycemia: excess of glucose in the blood – as seen in diabetes mellitus

Hyperlipidemia: increased levels of fats or lipids in the blood – increasing the risk of disease of the blood vessels leading to stroke and heart disease

Hypertension: blood pressure is higher than 140 over 90 mmHg
Hypertrophy: enlargement resulting from an increase in the size of cells
Hypotensive: abnormally low blood pressure
Hypothalamic: relating to the hypothalamus – the hypothalamus controls the pituitary gland and regulates many body functions
Incident: An incident is an occurrence of something that is often unpleasant
Inflammation: a complex biological response of body tissues to harmful stimuli
Inotropic: increasing or decreasing the force of muscular contractions – a positive heart inotropic agent increases the force of contraction; a negative ionotropic agent, the reverse
Insomnia: difficulty in falling or staying asleep
Insulin resistance: inability of the body cells to respond to insulin effectively, often leading to high blood sugar.
Interleukin-6: an endogenous chemical which is active in inflammation
Intima: the innermost layer of a blood vessel
Intracranial: within the skull
Intravenous: situated within, performed within, occurring within, or administered by entering a vein (intravenously)
Immune function: the response of the immune system to protect the body – when threatened by foreign substances, cells, and tissue
Ischemia: in cardiology usually referred to a shortage of blood and oxygen to the heart muscle – often resulting from a narrowing or blockage of the coronary arteries
Ischemic heart disease: heart disease due to ischemia – usually due to atherosclerosis
Lactose: a disaccharide (sugar) present in milk – some people are lactose intolerant and develop symptoms such as bloating and diarrhea on drinking milk
Lipid: fatty acids, oils, waxes, sterols, and triglycerides – they are insoluble in water
Lipoprotein: a particle that is the primary mean of transport of cholesterol and triglycerides in the blood
LDL: low density lipoprotein – the 'bad' cholesterol
Macrophages: large white blood cells in the tissues or blood – they engulf foreign substances or invaders such as cellular debris, foreign substances, microbes, cancer cells
Macular degeneration: deterioration of the small central area of the retina of the eye that controls visual acuity
Marfan's syndrome: a genetic disorder affecting the body's connective tissue

Mediterranean: referring to the Mediterranean Sea or the lands surrounding it

METs: A metabolic unit used to quantify the intensity of physical activity - commonly used in stress testing of the heart

Meta-analysis: a quantitative statistical analysis of several separate but similar experiments or studies – the pooled data usually provides more precise conclusions

Metabolic Syndrome: the co-occurrence of several known cardiovascular risk factors, including insulin resistance, obesity, atherogenic dyslipidemia and hypertension

Minerals: naturally occurring inorganic compounds

Mitral valve prolapse: a condition in which the leaflets of the mitral valve bulge (prolapse) into the heart's left upper chamber (left atrium) when the heart contracts

Monosaccharides: a class of sugars that cannot be broken down to simpler sugars

Monounsaturated: A fatty acid chain is monounsaturated if it contains one double bond

Myocardial Infarction: a heart attack – resulting from an abrupt stoppage of blood flow to the heart and causing heart muscle damage

NEPA: non-exercise physical activity

Neuro-hormonal: a hormone produced by or acting on nervous tissue – examples: acetylcholine or norepinephrine

Nicotine: the chief active constituent of tobacco – an addictive alkaloid

Nitric oxide: a major vasodilator

Noradrenaline: norepinephrine – a neurotransmitter that constricts blood vessels, raising blood pressure and heart rate and dilates bronchi of the lungs

Nor-epinephrine: noradrenaline - a neurotransmitter that constricts blood vessels, raising blood pressure and heart rate and dilates bronchi of the lungs

Obstructive sleep apnea: a serious breathing disorder – the throat muscles intermittently relax and block the airway during sleep

Oligosaccharides: a saccharide containing a small number (typically two to ten) of simple sugars (monosaccharides).

Omega 3: essential fatty acids found in fish oils, that help to lower the levels of cholesterol and LDL (low-density lipoproteins) in the blood.

Omega 6: long-chain polyunsaturated fatty acids, such as linoleic acid and arachidonic acid

Orthostatic: relating to or caused by erect posture

Osteoporosis: increased bone weakness from loss of bone mineral density increasing the risk of fractures

Oxidation: the process or result of oxidizing

Oxidative stress: imbalance between the production of free radicals and the ability of the body to counteract or detoxify their harmful effects

Parasympathetic: part of the autonomic nervous system that controls equilibrium of the physiological processes of the body at rest - the "rest and digest" function.

Pathogenesis: the biological mechanism that leads to the development of a disease

Percutaneous coronary intervention

Periodontal: supporting structures of the teeth including the gums, cementum, periodontal membranes, and alveolar bone.

Peripheral: situated away from the center

Peripheral artery disease: narrowing of the peripheral arteries, usually the leg arteries - due to atherosclerosis

Peroxidation: rancidity from oxidative deterioration of lipids

Phenols: A simple cyclic compound in fruits and green tea which is cardioprotective

Phobia: a persistent, abnormal, or irrational fear of a specific thing or situation

Phytochemicals: naturally occurring, plant based chemicals, that are biologically active and beneficial to our health.

Phytonutrients: plant based compounds that have health-protecting qualities

Phytosterols: sterols derived from plants. When consumed, they help block cholesterol absorption, resulting in a reduction of the blood cholesterol levels

Pituitary: a pea sized endocrine gland attached to the brain – it produces hormones that control other *glands*

Placebo: a harmless pill, medicine, or procedure

Plaque: atherosclerotic lesion within the wall of an artery that causes its inner lining to bulge into the lumen

Plaque vulnerability: the vulnerability of an atherosclerotic vessel plaque to rupture or cause the formation of a blood clot in the vessel – may lead to a myocardial infarction or sudden death.

Platelets: a small, round, thin blood cells that circulate through our bloodstream. Their role is to help stop bleeding

Polyphenols: naturally occurring plant compounds with antioxidant activity that prevents or neutralizes the damaging effects of free radicals.

Polysaccharides: long chains of monosaccharide units bound together by glycosidic linkages – examples are starch, glycogen, and cellulose

Polycystic ovary syndrome: a hormonal disorder in women that can affect their periods, ovulation, fertility and pregnancy.

Polyunsaturated: A fatty acid chain is *polyunsaturatea* if it contains more than one double bond.

Postmenopausal: after menopause

Postprandial glucose: blood sugar after eating a meal, usually after 1 and 2 hours

Prehypertension: blood pressure between 120/80 mmHg and 139/89 mmHg

Premature: occurring before the expected time

Premenstrual syndrome: a wide variety of complex symptoms experienced by some women prior to *menstruation*

Prevalence: proportion of a population that is affected with a particular disease at a given time.

Primary prevention: to prevent disease or injury before it occurs

Prophylactic: preventive

Prothrombotic: increasing the risk of thrombosis (developing a blood clot in a blood vessel)

PTSD: Post Traumatic Stress Disorder

Pulmonary: relating to the lungs

Quintile: used in statistics - where the sample or population is divided into fifths

Randomized: make unpredictable; in a clinical trial, people are allocated by chance to receive one of several clinical interventions

Revascularization: to restore blood flow – usually by vascular bypass and angioplasty

Ribonucleic acid: RNA - acts as a messenger between DNA and the protein synthesis complexes, called ribosomes

Saturated fats: saturated fats have no double bonds because they are saturated with hydrogen molecules. Saturated fats are typically solid at room temperature.

Schizophrenia: a chronic and severe mental disorder which affects how a person thinks, feels and acts.

Secondary prevention: to stop or slow the progression of a disease or injury already established

Snuff: smokeless tobacco made from ground or pulverized tobacco leaves

Statins: a group of cholesterol lowering drugs

Stroke: cutting off blood flow to a part of the brain resulting in permanent damage

Supplement: a product taken orally that contains one or more ingredients, such as vitamins or amino acids to add further nutritional value

Sympathetic nervous system: A part of the autonomic nervous system that accelerates the heart rate, constricts blood vessels, and raises blood pressure – the fight or flight response.

Systolic blood pressure: pressure your blood is exerting against your artery walls when the heart beats. If the blood pressure is 120/80, the systolic pressure is 120 mm Hg (millimeters of mercury).

Therapeutic: healing/curing; relating to the treatment of disease

Thermogenesis: heat production by metabolic processes; the process of energy production in the body

Thrombosis: the formation of a blood clot inside a blood vessel

Thrombotic: pertaining to thrombosis

Thrombus: a blood clot within a blood vessel

Tobacco: dried leaves of this plant - smoked in cigarettes, pipes, or cigars, or chewed

Tocopherols: organic chemical compounds with vitamin E antioxidant activity

Transcendental meditation: silent *meditation using a mantra* and other yogic practices

Transient ischemic attack: a mini-stroke, usually lasting only a few minutes and causing no permanent damage

Trans-fat: artificially created by adding hydrogen to liquid vegetable oils to make them more solid

Triglycerides: lipids that are esters formed from one molecule of glycerol and three molecules of one or more fatty acids They are stored in the fat cells and are a major source of energy in the body.

Unsaturated fats: a *fat* or fatty acid in which there is at least one double bond within the fatty acid chain – these are healthier than saturated fats

Unstable angina: angina due to inadequate blood flow to the heart that may lead to a myocardial infarction.

Vasoconstriction: the narrowing/constriction of the blood vessels

Vasomotor: relating to the caliber of the blood vessels (constriction or dilatation)

Vasospasm: spasm of a blood vessel – constriction which may lead to the restriction of blood flow

Ventricular arrhythmias: Abnormal rapid heart rhythms originating in the ventricles of the heart

Visceral: relating to the inner organs of the body

Vitamin: group of organic compounds required by the body in small amounts for proper functioning and growth

ABOUT THE AUTHOR

Neil K. Agarwal, MD is presently doing his third-year clinical residency in Internal Medicine at Drexel University/Hahneman University Hospital in Philadelphia, PA. He completed his undergraduate studies in biomedical engineering at Rutgers University, New Brunswick, NJ. He obtained his medical degree from St. George's University School of Medicine in Grenada, West Indies in 2015. He has been active in volunteering work both locally and internationally. He has travelled to Hondurus and Panama to help in medical clinics in the past. He has been active in clinical research and has presented over 30 abstracts/posters at several national and international scientific meetings and has published over 10 articles in peer reviewed medical journals.

Shashi K. Agarwal, MD is a retired Cardiologist. He graduated from Grant Medical College, Bombay University, India in 1974. He was the Chief Medical Resident at Bergen Pines County Hospital in Paramus, New Jersey in 1979. He finished his Cardiology Fellowship from the University of New Mexico School of Medicine and Affiliated Hospitals in 1981. Dr. Agarwal obtained his Board Certification in Internal Medicine in 1979 and Cardiovascular Diseases in 1981. He had been a Fellow of the American College of Physicians, American College of Cardiology and the American College of Chest Physicians. He has presented over 150 scientific abstracts/posters at both national and international scientific meetings and has published over 50 full length medical articles in peer reviewed medical journals.

hearthealthylifestyles@gmail.com